# LOVE

## Learning Of Various Epidemics

***Teaching Students and Communities how to live a Safer and Healthier Lifestyle***

**Evern Vinson Williams**

**An American Pioneer**

## DEDICATION PAGE

I dedicate this book to my son Evern Leland Williams and my Mother Ms. Angelo Williams, your presence and spirit from God has truly been a blessing and motivation for me.

And to all the Graduates of 2020, for your courage, strength and endurance and determination to finish the drill despite it all! Also, to the victims and families of the world who have lost loved ones from Covid-19. May you let your light always shine to inspire others.

# CONTENT

# ACKNOWLEDGMENT

*I have learned a lot from my experiences and from the support of others. My acknowledgements are first to GOD for allowing me to utilize a unique gift in a way to benefit mankind. My mother Angelo Williams who continues to push me to higher endeavors and who began teaching and training me way before schools. To my brothers and sisters Priscilla, Linda, Eddie, Eric, and Edward for your unyielding support. To My better half, Ms. Leann Johnson for your enduring motivation and encouragement.*

*To the late, Dr. Stephen B. Thacker ret. US, for your leadership and belief in my ability to create and lead. It is through your determined spirit this book was driven. Dr. David Kleinbaum for your support and guidance as a novel distinguished professor of epidemiology. The late, Frank Snowball Smith, a mentor that has always shown support for all within his community.*

# 1

# Beginning Journey

I have always been taught that education was the key to success. From a child growing up in Detroit Michigan, education has been an especially important aspect of my life. I was blessed at birth to have both my mother and my father. As a young toddler, I remember waking up every Saturday morning watching Soul Train with my dad. This was a tradition that my father and I did every Saturday morning. After Soul Train if he were not going fishing with his cousins, uncles and my older brothers, he would take me riding with him in his pickup work truck to collect scrap metal.

My father was always a hard worker and a man of many constructive talents. Welding, framing, building mechanics, metal scrap collector, fisherman, and grill master. A natural entrepreneur, always having a side job to make ends meet to provide for his family. My dad was also an incredibly talented man and began driving large 18-wheeler trucks at the young age of 16 back in Montgomery Alabama in 1961. This was odd for a young black male in the early 60's to drive an 18-wheeler truck but he wasn't the normal 16-year-old young man. Always creative, witty, and seem to understand how hard work pays off. He quit school at the age of 15 and began working full time.

By the time he was 17 years of age he purchased his first vehicle and was one of only a few young black teenagers in his community to purchase a vehicle. He was always creating new ways to do things. My mother and father had 4 children in Montgomery Alabama in the 60's, two boys and two girls. After the Civil Rights Movement, there were a growing number of industrial jobs in the north. Both my mother and dad decided to move to Detroit Michigan in 1969. I was born a year later followed by my younger brother Edward in Detroit Michigan. We were given the nicknames "Yankees" of the family because we were born up north! We still laugh about this till this day: always wearing the sign of the north. I wore it proudly because I was born in a different place!

Our family values were quite simple. My father was the provider and worked sometimes 7 days a week while my mom worked just as hard taking care of all six children at home. Family and close friends were always close to him. A small framed man with a huge personality.

I remember my two older brothers going with my dad on fishing trips while I had to stay at home with mama and my younger brother. I asked him if I could go on the trips and he told me when I turned 7 years of age. I was so excited the closer it got to my seventh birthday which was on April 12, 1977. Each month and day gave me more excitement and joy. I would say "I am going fishing in a few months" to my brothers and sisters. On the morning of March 8, 1977 my father said, "I'll see you later cat". Unfortunately, these turned out to be the last words I heard him say.

My father was killed on his job. I remember thinking this could not really be happening. Yet it did. That day and his spirit has always reminded me of how quick life has a way of altering your plans. The strongest part of my shield and which allowed me to get through all the pain was the love of family and friends growing up. At the age of 6, I learned how valuable life was and how quick it can be taken away from you.

Later in life, this passion would transfer. I researched fatal occupational injuries as an ever-increasing epidemic. There were no regulations holding employers accountable for providing a safe environment for employees at the time. While the 1970 Occupational Safety and Health Act was established to regulate safety for workers and to reduce work related accidents and deaths, more than 6,500 people still die yearly in the U.S. due to accidental/occupational related deaths. See *http://www.ajc.com/news/traffic/worker-killed-crash-construction-site-driver-believed-*impaired/FJZ8Ff5AWSUBVQQHNsANuJ/.

My first experience losing someone due to an epidemic. A decline in this number did not occur until 2011. So, the history of today, tells us that 6 to 7 thousand people die each year on their jobs, except for the year 2011 when this number dipped to 4600. The US Department of Labor Statistics reported the phenomena by state.

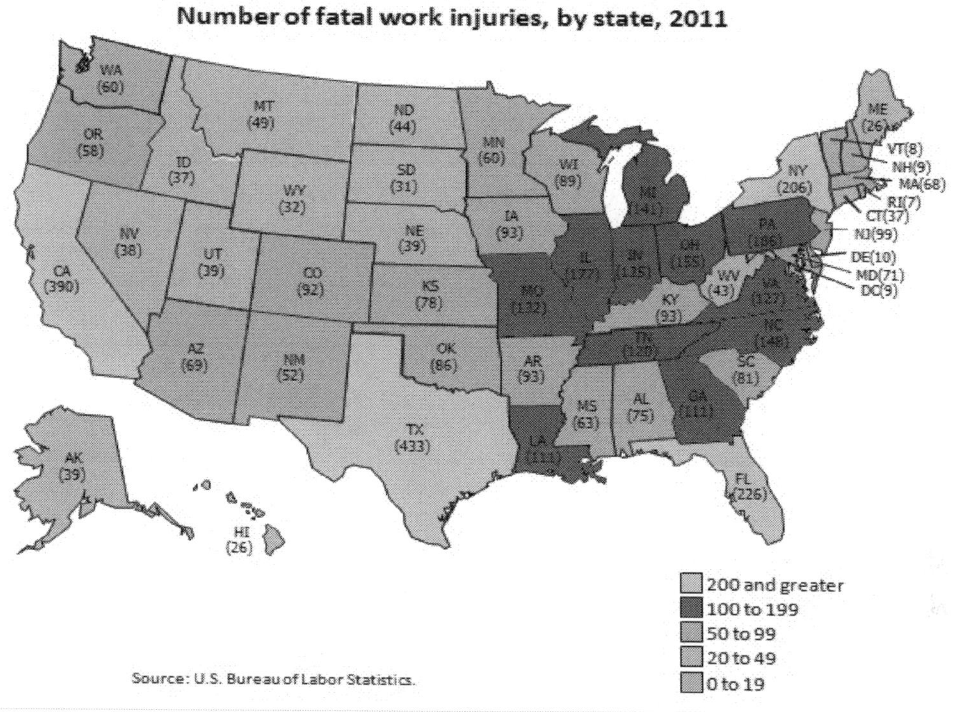


https://www.bls.gov/opub/btn/volume-2/death-on-the-job-fatal-work-injuries-in-2011.htm

Although my father died before I was able to go enjoy the fishing trip. I was thankful for knowing and hearing some of the stories of his life. Several of these stories allows me to understand more about myself.

My father once purchased a car with no gas tank in it. Apparently, he needed to get the car home (Guess, getting it towed was not an option). He ran a tube from the engine into a five-gallon gas container that was placed on the floor of the passenger seat. He managed to drive it back to the house. If you are a student reading this book, please do not try this at home. I was told and by his brothers that he had the gift of gab, a natural comedian and a fancy dresser. He was even given the nickname 'Dance Machine'. The apple does not fall far from the tree! Thankful to GOD for the time I was able to spend with my dad. While I lean on his legacy, my mother's persistence, determination and courage was the foundation of my life.

Shortly after daddy died, I remember mama enrolling into night school and taking a part time job during the day. As a child, I would watch her fight to stay awake after class to help me and my brothers and sisters with homework. It was obvious that she valued and was dedicated to education. We never wore the latest name brands, but we were neat and clean. Mama taught us that appearance reflected on the type of person you were.

I will never forget the first holiday season after my father's death. Thanksgiving was spaghetti and meatballs while watching the Detroit Lions football team on television. The tradition of watching the Lions made the experience somewhat normal but daddy's absence made a big difference. It was simple. Mama did not feel like cooking. Christmas was a drive down south to visit mother's side of the family in Montgomery Alabama. The car broke down in Ohio on the way back during a snowstorm. Mom made sure we were safe and warm with blankets in our yellow 1973 Buick. Lucky for us, our uncle Buddy lived in Ohio and was close enough to drive us back to Detroit.

Mama did her best, providing unconditional love to six children. Family was always considered first. She provided us a canvas of her life meant to be followed. While working and completing night nursing school she always found a way to make it work. Her motto was always 'do what you got to do', and "time waits for no one".

I was introduced to science classes early in life. I remember mama meeting my younger brother and I at the elementary school to catch the bus with her to attend nursing classes at night. From McFarland Elementary school we went downtown Detroit Michigan. We sat in the back of the classroom and were trained to stay quiet. Mama never had to say a word. When she raised one eyebrow with her eyes opened wide, we knew to stop whatever we were doing and to get the behavior right. We even called ourselves taking notes in her Anatomy class and would come home and compare our notes with mamas. Always putting her children first and finding a way to move forward is just one of her characteristics.

Mama would always discuss with us the different aspects of her duties and responsibilities as a nurse's aide. She also did her homework while we did ours in the same area. It was both her words and actions that was a constant reminder of the importance of education. Working as a Certified Nursing Assistant, I remember her telling me the number of people that were severely ill with life threatening illnesses. They were not able to take a shower or even go to the restroom without assistance. I asked mom if she was responsible for making sure they were clean after doing number 2? Number two was known then as a description of a bile movement. Her response was "yes" with a smile. I thought to myself that was something I would not look forward to doing. She was dedicated, determined and persistent in her relentless battle to support six children as a widowed mother. My mom always had a natural love and service for those who were sick. She would sometimes describe how several of her patients were dying from some form of cancer.

And would always tell me how cancer was a deadly disease that kills all types of people in America. Discussing health issues openly and honestly with all of us was a common characteristic of my mother.

Somehow, I believe she saw death so much that she became numb to the emotions of patients dying. With most of her patients suffering from stage 4 cancer, my mother stressed the emphasis of living a healthy lifestyle to avoid future health risk. I remember her constantly discussing and describing the different diseases and the short- and long-term effects of the illness.

She described cancer as a disease in which abnormal cells are rapidly produced that do not function as normal tissue within an organ. Mama would always describe the known cause and effects of diseases. I remember her telling us that back in the day, during the 60's and early 70's smoking was one of the coolest things to do. It was a socially acceptable habit from all cultures. It was even lawful for teachers to smoke in the teachers' lounge. No one knew at the time the dangers associated with such actions. The long-term effects of smoking were not a primary concern at the time. Currently, one of the single most-deadliest killer epidemics in the U.S. is cigarettes. Responsible for more than 600,000 deaths a year in the U. S. alone according to statistics. It is highly addictive and known to cause lung cancer and increase hypertension in the body My mom had to raise 6 children on her own and making sure we had what we needed and not getting sick was one of her primary concerns. Therefore, she constantly always gave good health advise and shared the good bad and the ugly of diseases. Currently, cancer kills more than 8.2 million people a year globally. Lung cancer causes more than 1.5 million deaths globally per year.

Allowing students to see and research the numbers of people affected by an epidemic give's students an idea of why this topic is important. On any given day anyone of us could fall victim to one of the several epidemics that causes severe illness throughout the world. One of my primary characteristics by students is that I keep it real by showing real numbers. Numbers do not lie and have a way of getting students attention. A chart such as the one below from the World Health Organization may be used to generate interest and discussions.

The World Health Organization lists the globe's leading types of cancers for 2018.

- Lung (2.09 million cases)
- Breast (2.09 million cases)
- Colorectal (1.80 million cases)
- Prostate (1.28 million cases)
- Skin cancer (non-melanoma) (1.04 million cases)
- Stomach (1.03 million cases)

The most common causes of cancer death are cancers of:

- Lung (1.76 million deaths)
- Colorectal (862 000 deaths)
- Stomach (783 000 deaths)
- Liver (782 000 deaths)
- Breast (627 000 deaths)

https://www.who.int/news-room/fact-sheets/detail/cancer

Prostate cancer is most dominate in black males. According to the Centers for Disease Control and Prevention, CDC, almost 20% of the black male population will develop prostate cancer. Cancer may be caused by a carcinogen, something that may cause or trigger normal cell development to become cancerous. Remembering my elementary school days most of the school buildings were covered with asbestos as it was the most widely used product to insulate and cover ceilings of most large buildings especially institutions of education. Fifteen years later, it became apparent that asbestos contained deadly carcinogens. As a result, over a period of ten years, all asbestos was removed from the ceilings of buildings nationwide. Most recently actor Chadwick Boseman died of colon cancer. What was shocking was that he was sick while filming the superhero movie "Black Panther. Mr. Boseman's speech at the commencement ceremony of Howard University for the class of 2018 was full of excitement, motivation and encouragement. His work in the film industry gave millions of Americans a superhero to be proud of.

My mother always stressed the importance of taking good care of your body. She could easily prepare us to protect ourselves from disease or infection. However, social epidemics became a problem in several of the minority communities in the mid 1970's. There were four boys and two girls in the home with my mother. Things began to change in the social behaviors of teenagers in the mid to late 70's. Between the years 1977 and 1978 I noticed more crimes beginning to emerge from teenagers. Students began to become more aggressive both in the schools and in the streets. My two oldest siblings attended McKenzie High School, the next two attended Drew

Junior High School, while my younger brother and I were in McFarland Elementary School.

One day after school, I witnessed one of my oldest brothers running home screaming one evening after getting off the bus. “Open the door Evern”, “Open the Door”! I did not know what to think until I saw a large crowd of teenagers running behind him. My brother quickly falls into the doorway on the porch as my sister and I quickly pushed the door shut and locked it. As my sister checked my brother to make sure he was alright, I took a quick peak out of the window to see a crowd of young men standing on the sidewalk gasping for breath and slamming their hands and fist together. At the time I could not understand what was going on but later learned that all those guys chasing my brother were gang members. They wanted an old leather jacket my brother was wearing, and they were willing to kill for it. I was scared and angry at the same time but knew that myself along with my sisters and brothers we were no match for a group of teenage boys. They soon left the house, and I could hear my brother and sister describing what happened to my mom as she entered the house. Two weeks later a student was stabbed to death at a local high school over a leather jacket. It was my first-time hearing of black on black homicide and it was a school within our school district in Detroit. Currently today black on black homicide is responsible for more than 75% of the deaths of black males between the age of 15 to 24 years of age. My mother went into protective mode. She decided to move back to Alabama where her family lived. Always making decisions ensuring the safety of her children.

# 2

# Growing Years

Moving from Detroit Michigan to Montgomery Alabama in the late 70's really gave me an eye opener at an early age. I think most can agree that there is a big difference between Detroit Michigan and Montgomery Alabama, yet my stereotypes of the south gave me more fear than the experience itself. I only imagined the south as the old movies and news clips of the civil rights movement, large fields with cows, segregation and racism. I did not know what to think, yet I knew it was time to leave Detroit with my family. I was excited and sad at the same time. Excited to be around my mom's side of the family yet sad to move to Alabama, far away from my father's side in Detroit and Chicago.

The south was very much different from the north. Beyond the stereotypes, the language was different. The word pop was no longer a part of the vocabulary as it was replaced with drank. While the word orange was changed to errrrng. Although there were some social differences, the people were much friendlier in the south. It was later bought to my attention that this is just a reflection of southern hospitality.

While my mother worked long shifts this left six children at home. Our sibling's age range was from 8 to 17 years of age. Regardless of what we were doing we knew that our mother had rules. Rules that did not bend with punishments given for those who did not follow them. Curfew was always nonnegotiable. The streetlight determined the time you were to come into the house. During the spring and summer months we enjoyed the extended time that daylight savings provided. My mom would always say, "Don't let the streetlight catch you". "When that streetlight comes on you need to be in the house or headed into the house". I can only imagine the number of nights that we talked to our friends in the neighborhood allowing the streetlight to come on and waiting to see if car lights were coming over the hill. It was nothing to be ashamed as all of us had a curfew. Once we saw headlights, we all took off running because we did not know if it was one of our parents driving home.

While growing up in the 80's I remember 4 major historical events. Ronald Reagan becoming the 38th President of the United States, Princess Diana's wedding to Prince Charles shown worldwide on television, famine relief in Ethiopia, Africa and the rise of AIDS, acquired Immune deficiency syndrome. These four topics dominated the media. We watched a lot of news, sports and shows that provided family entertainment. There was no VCR, Microwave, Internet, cell phone, pager, or YouTube. "Happy Days", "Dukes of Hazards", "The incredible Hulk", Soul Train, "Good Times", "Mr. Rogers", "Sesame Street", and "Dallas" were the shows I watched growing up as young child. As a teenager "The Cosby Show", "Good Times and "The Jefferson's" were some of my favorites. The Price is Right, Jeopardy, Family Feud, and let me not forget Days of Our

Lives, Young and the Restless and Another World! I never thought at the time how these shows made such an impact on my upbringing. Everyone wanted that Cosby show family and the Claire Huxtable wife. A black male doctor on television with a black wife who was a lawyer. This was the first television show that depicted both black parents as academically successful. Looking back at it now, I realized that so many of my friends and peers were influenced in a positive way by this show. How much of an influence did television and radio have on shaping my life and ambitions? How much influence does social media have on the behaviors of our children today? Today social media and television plays a major role in the influence or our youth. Growing up in the south was nothing like I thought at least in Montgomery Alabama.

It took some time for me to get adjusted to the school system in the south. I realized the culture was different. Yes, Sir and No Sir were words used to respond to questions asked by adults. In the south this is seen as a sign of respect. However, in the north it was considered old historical language reflecting days of slavery and hierarchy within a culture. I remember my mom attending parent conferences for all of us at some point because one or more of us would not say "yes mam" and "yes sir" to a teacher. We were taught to say yes "Mr. Smith" instead of yes sir. My mom won that battle quick as she did not back down easy.

Chisholm Elementary School was the first public school I attended in Montgomery Alabama in 1978. The school was predominately white with most students receiving free and reduced lunch. My mother later transferred us to Fews Elementary school so that our grandmother could supervise us while she worked various shifts. Fews happen to be my mother and father's alma matter elementary school with a majority black population. I was a student who was a little different from most. I made good grades but took little time to develop patience with students who tried to bully me because of my small statue and size. I remember in 1982 while attending Fews Elementary school I was an honor roll student, yet I was suspended 6 times in one year for fighting. In every incident I was being bullied so I was never kicked out of school, instead I was admitted back in after a parent conference. I remember my last fight, Mr. Mack the acting assistant principal at the time, decided that my punishment would be 3 licks with the paddle. I looked up at this man as he was more than 6 feet 8 inches tall and weighed close to 300 lbs. I remember thinking, he had to be a former football lineman or something. Mr. Mack stood over me and sat the paddle on the desk and asked me to stand up. Suddenly his radio began to beep as he received a call to the front office at the time. He said "I'll be back and proceeded out of his office and closed the door, leaving me in his office alone with the paddle on the desk. I began thinking this man is about to hit me with this paddle. I immediately noticed the light shining through his small windows about 6 feet above the ground. crawled up on his desk and began to climb the wall and opened the window. Jumping out the window and landing safely on the ground, I began running as fast as I could across the field into a local neighborhood. I could hear Mr. Mack screaming in the background, "Hey Evern, come back". The more he yelled my name, the faster I would run. I knew eventually they would get in their cars and come to look for me, so I decided to enter an abandoned apartment building. I could hear the administrators and police outside looking for me. I saw the string to the attic of an abandoned apartment and decided to hide in this area until the search calmed down. Patiently waiting for the search to stop I had to sit in this attic for hours while they continued their search even as far as walking directly under me in this abandoned apartment. Once the search calmed down, I decided to sneak my way home hiding while watching those looking for me and going unnoticed during my journey through the back yards of all the neighbor's house until I got home. I remember walking into the house while my mother was on the phone with the school. She was disappointed that Mr. Mack threatened to paddle me and for not providing the proper safety at school, allowing me to get lost. As I entered the back door of my great grandmothers' home, my mother looked at me and immediately told them "he is right here". They could not believe it as they looked for me for hours and was still surveying the area with police trying to look for me. My mother was happy to see me, yet she did get on to me about hiding in an abandoned apartment. After telling her how I got home she laughed and was amazed at how I did not get caught by any of them. I left the six-grade with honors.

After elementary school I attended Bellingrath Junior High School. Most of my friends from elementary school attended other middle schools and some did not make it to middle school at all or went to juvenile before middle school. It was then I began to get involved in extracurricular activities. I ran cross country track, played soccer and was a first seat all city trumpet player. My brother Edward and I also participated in several science fairs and received several academic scholastic and leadership awards. My sports days were not long lasting as I was not able to play football since my mom thought I was too small in junior high to play a contact sport. Seems she made a good decision for me since the latest research shows head injuries for so many former football players. Soccer happened to be my most recognized sport as I was MVP in Junior High. It was my first-time playing soccer. My position was center, and I played it with the best of my ability. I also played the position of center field and pitcher on one of the city little league baseball teams. I was selected to play on the Montgomery City All-star team as a center fielder. I remember riding the bench in the all-star game and not getting a chance to play unless we had a large lead. I knew I was the smallest of them all, but I was faster than all those bigger boys. After the season I never cared to play organized baseball again. Finishing up junior High school I began preparing to go to a 6A powerhouse high school that had a reputation for being the best high school within the city in both scholastic academic and athletic accomplishments.

Robert E. Lee High School was the name of my high school. I was in the marching, symphony, and jazz band playing trumpet and bass guitar. As a student in a classroom, I must admit the most exciting times were my extracurricular activities, science labs and band. School for the most part seemed simple and easy as I was always motivated by classes in which there was interaction with other students. During my senior year I took an art class as an elective in which I won 1st place in a major city art contest. I always had a natural gift as an artist, yet I never put enough time in growing my art, as I consider it as a gift that allows me to have mental relaxation and expression.

Growing up I never thought of becoming a teacher. A policeman, fireman, artist, medical doctor, or athlete were just a few of the careers that I aspired to become. Teaching was the furthest thing from my mind.

While in high school one of my sisters Linda worked as an optical Lab Technician for an eye doctor in Tuskegee Alabama. During the summer months before band season started, I would visit Dr. Bells office and shadow his position as an optometrist. I enjoyed the experience but did not think I was getting enough interaction. I knew if not an optometrist, some type of medical doctor or sports medicine physician would be a career that seemed to fit my passion. I enjoyed working with people and science. At the time during the 80's if you were passionate about science, you were either a medical doctor or nurse. None of the other careers seemed to provide a guaranteed favorable job market. Furthermore, there were no mention of other health careers in public health.

Robert E. Lee along with the rebel flag was the mascots of our high school. I remember the large life-sized brass sculpture of Robert E. Lee standing directly in front of the school. A school filled with all cultures. At the time, no one complained or challenged the mascot. I never thought to ask why this was our mascot because I knew who the mascot represented as well as the history. However, everyone was almost subconsciously accepting what was provided which was a free public education regardless of the name of the school. Therefore, I do not remember any issues with the name of the school as a community issue. Currently within the media there are several facilities across the country considering renaming mascots and names representing specific reflections of history that may be offensive to various cultures. I guess every generation has a level of acceptance when it comes to what they feel is offensive, justice or injustice. Or could it be that social media has provided an avenue to obtain knowledge that has now influenced our behavior? Two weeks ago, the statue of Robert E. Lee was removed from my old alma matter. And recently several monuments representing the confederacy or support of slavery have been removed from across the country. I never would have expected this to happen after I finished my book, but it did. The year of 2020 has been a year of surprises and revelations. I graduated in 1988 at the top percent of my class and was blessed to receive a band scholarship from Troy State University in Troy Alabama.

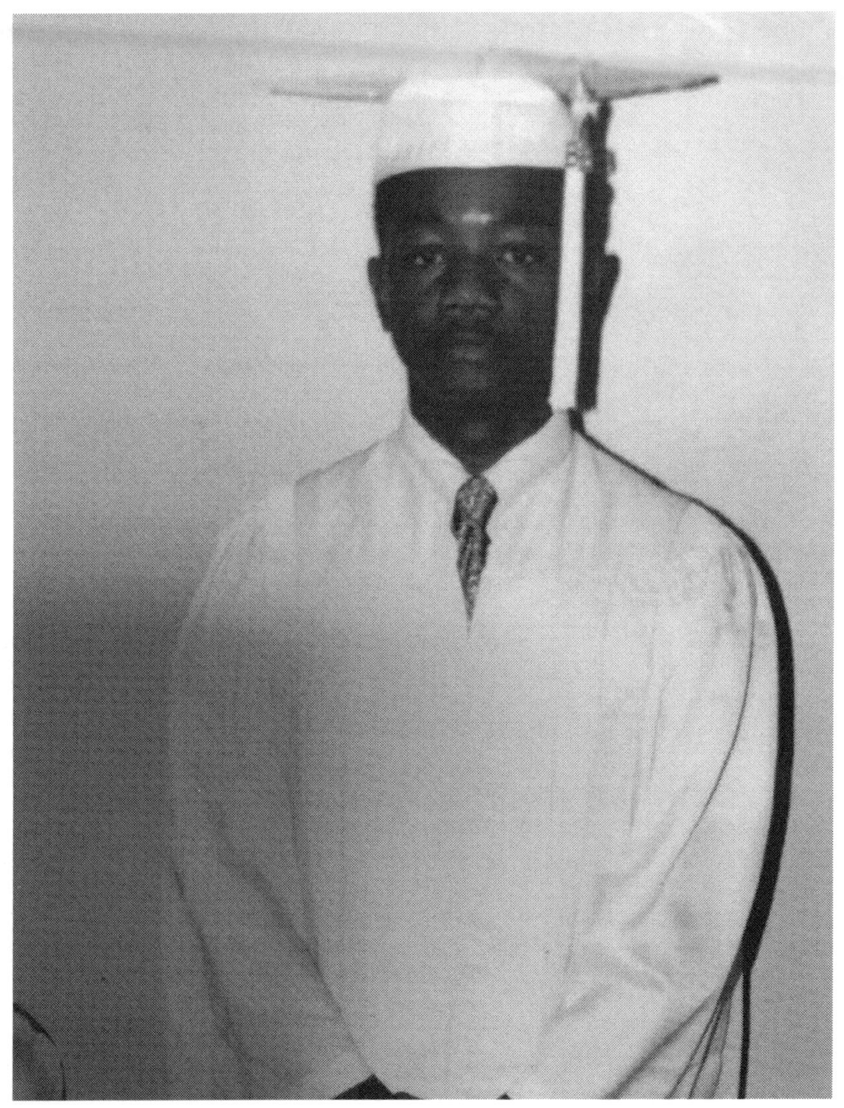

# 3

# College Days

I attended Troy State University, under a band scholarship. My major was Pre-Med as I was planning to become an optometrist. While in college, I participated in several activities. Playing the trumpet for the Troy State University Band in 1988, was a distinct honor to me as Dr. John M. Long the band director was a legend known for his talents as a well-known and established band director. Our band was known as the Sound of the South and used the well-known song as Dixie every time we marched off the field. For the record, it did not bother me at all to play this song I was more focused on getting the notes and the glide step while marching off the field. At the time, African Americans made up about 10% of the population of students on campus. We were all awfully close and always knew of one another at least the full-time students who lived on or off campus. I participated in several intramural sports including football, and basketball. I pledged and joined Kappa Psi, a band service fraternity in 1989. My brother Eric was already a member of the fraternity and yes, he initiated me with others into the brotherhood. Our chapter, Zeta Upsilon was unique from some of our nearby brothers from HBCU's, Alabama State University and Tuskegee University. Our membership was mixed with both black, white, asian and latino members. I remember attending my first Kappa Kappa Psi district convention with all the brothers from various chapters within the southeastern states. After the business meetings, and during the social time fraternity brothers from the HBCU's would host step shows against one another. North Carolina A&T, Alabama State University, Tuskegee University, Florida A&M University and Bethune Cookman. After watching their performance, I stated to my brothers Eric and Andre Burgess, I want to step like these brothers on our campus. Our chapter never stepped and at the time we had about 8 African American Brothers and 20 White Brothers. Andre' Burgess and I stayed outside with the brothers from Bethune Cookman and learned the fundamentals of stepping with traditional steps such as "Groovie" and "Loose Neck" from the hours of 11:00 pm to 6:00 am the next morning in the parking lot of the hotel room.

After returning to campus, we suggested to get a step team within our chapter, Zeta Upsilon, Troy University. Some of the brothers looked at us as if we were crazy but we were determined and persistent. Within a few weeks we had our first Kappa Kappa Psi step team on the campus of Troy University. At the beginning only the African American brothers stepped at the step shows. We began with six steppers and would compete against the other fraternities on campus during Greek Show Step competitions. It was uncommon for nonsocial fraternities to step in a step show. We stepped in our first Greek Show on Campus and won second place only to our brothers from Alabama State University. They stepped with more than 21 brothers and really deserved to win as they had so many synchronized steppers performing an exceptionally good show.

For the next few years, we would always win second place at any step show we competed in. I remember after missing first place by the same team we decided to get several of our nonblack brothers to step with us. They were percussionist, or horn players and knew how rhythm and sounds work together. I figured I could teach them how to step and really shock a predominately black audience who had never seen white brothers' step in their life. We practiced more than 30 hours a week for months preparing for our shows. And for this one, we worked even harder as we wanted to win and beat our brothers from Alabama State University. Not only was our chapters close in proximity we were also close in brotherhood. Regardless of the color of your skin we were brothers as music was a common factor in our brotherhood. We all had something in common. We depended on one another during our pledging days. White and black brothers who knew little about one another were taught and forced to depend on one another for support. I can tell you joining this organization was one of the most influential aspects of shaping my opinions, thoughts and learning how we are all the same. I later joined Alpha Phi Alpha fraternity incorporated in 1991. I learned more from this organization and other social fraternities the importance of community service and the impact one group may have on those who need it most. I remember stepping at a step show with both organizations. I think I was one of the first people to step in the same step show as the step master for two fraternities competing in the same Greek show. Every organization has their own style of stepping within the Panhellenic organizations. I stepped against the Alphas before I was an Alpha with the Kappa Kappa Psi brothers in the past. My Alpha Brothers wanted to know if I was stepping with Kappa Kappa Psi, I told them yes. So, they understood that I was stepping with both organizations. There were about 12 other Greek Fraternity's competing in this show from Tuskegee, Alabama A&M, Alabama State and Florida A&M University. The Kappa Kappa Psi brothers from Alabama State also competed in this show. I stepped with both of my fraternities as we won 1st and 2nd place in the same step show. During the show I can remember when we surprised the crowed by revealing all our white brothers to a culture that had never seen white boys' step before. It was an epic event as they began dancing and stepping from the back of the auditorium through the aisles of several hundred students screaming and cheering for them. When they joined us on stage no one could tell the brothers apart as all our steps sounds and rhythm patterns were precise and accurate as we were all in the marching band. We also had the numbers to be more creative and impressive as we were stepping with more than 18 fraternity brothers. We won the step show while my Alpha brothers that I stepped with about an hour earlier won second place. I could not believe that I was a part of two fraternities that won 1st and second place in the same step show with competitors from our neighboring HBCU schools. Everyone was happy for the brothers as we all celebrated together on the campus of Troy University after the Greek Show. I graduated in 1992 with my Bachelor of Science degree in Biology minoring in Chemistry and

Physics. I thank those who were able to begin breaking the chains of segregation so that I was able to accomplish my goal. To know that the late Mr. John Lewis began his fight for equal rights with Troy University, opened my eyes to more of my purpose within this world. John Lewis was denied entrance in the late 50's into Troy State. Before civil rights or integration of schools. He was given the name "That boy from Troy" by Dr. Martin Luther. King. I now consider myself "Just another Boy From Troy".

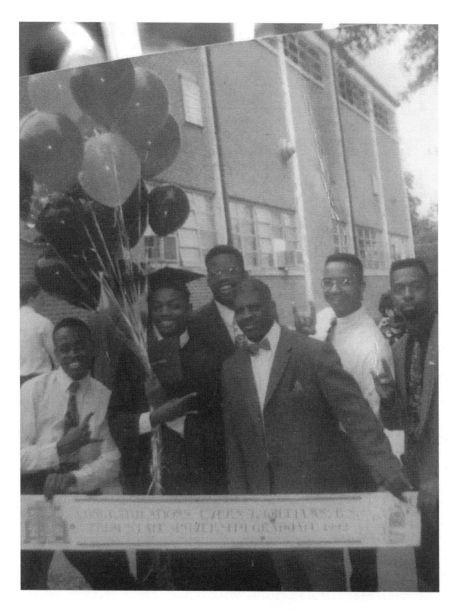

After receiving my B.S. in biology, I still was not sure of where to go so decided to pursue my master's degree at Troy. I served as microbiology lab supervisor for most of my undergraduate years. Before receiving my B. S. Dr. Chapman asked me if I was interested in teaching some of the microbiology labs. I was shocked and really honored that he asked me as I always found my lab job interesting.

Keeping up with the cultures in the media prep area was one thing but to teach a class of college students was something I looked forward too.

. Yes, I stood out like a sore thumb, as a black male teaching science at Troy University. I would say it was a combination of both my talents and timing. I began teaching microbiology, Anatomy and Botany labs at Troy University at the beginning of my first graduate year of college. My professors, Dr. Chapman, Dr. Woods, and Mrs. Kean, all gave me the opportunity to teach labs for each of their classes within the same semester. So, there I was 22-year-old black male teaching upper level science labs for aspiring nurses, doctors and other future health care professionals at Troy University a predominately white college in 1992. As you can imagine, several students attempted to challenge both my intellectual and professional abilities as a lab instructor. Younger than most of the students in the classroom, and being black, I focused on professionalism and maintained barriers for conversations. It was not long before all the students in the classroom realized that I was not intimidated by my age, or the fact that I was the only black instructor within the science department. I do not know if they were impressed, shocked or really thrown off to see this person who was still finishing up an undergraduate degree teach labs to college students with no previous teaching experience.

My professors stated that I was a naturally gifted instructor who knew how to address issues with an ability to disseminate information in an interesting and unique way. One thing I realized with teaching from the very beginning, is that everybody has their own strengths and weaknesses. I recognized my weaknesses first before I could Identify my strengths.

I will say that I focused on teaching students how to learn, understand and apply relevant information in a way to solve real world problems Teachers were underpaid and overworked in my mind therefore a career in it wasn't an option for me.

During my teaching experience at Troy State University I realized more and more that teaching was more of a gift for me and not a job. It was enjoyable. With my college students I focused on making sure I connected my student's curriculum with accurate and relevant information. The students learned more how to break down information so that it was understandable. While describing a gram stain to college students, I would push to indicate the importance of isolating bacteria cultures and how that relates to the advancement of medical breakthroughs. I began gaining lots of positive attention with my teaching strategies and was being recognized and recruited by other professors to teach their labs. Later teaching Anatomy & Physiology and Botany labs.

A few months before finishing graduate school I did not know exactly what I wanted to pursue as a career. I only knew that teaching did not feel like work for me. At the time, teaching felt more of a hobby instead of a career. It was relaxing to give someone the gift of knowledge and watch their eyes and face transform as they begin to understand something. Or the fact that several of my students would stay after a lecture in college and further discuss the topics with me after class not wanting to end the lecture. I realized as I excelled in teaching that maybe I should stay in this field for just a little bit longer.

I decided to attend the teacher recruitment held at the university. While visiting different school systems, I meet a noticeably short older gentleman with a personality of gold. He talked about his sons, his wife, and his town. I was impressed with his story lines and conversation. He was an absolute comedian with a personality that would keep anyone laughing. Dr. Julian Cope was the superintendent of schools for Jasper County Schools in Monticello Georgia. He was one of the few superintendents attending the jobs fair and that caught my attention as he was reluctant in his way of recruiting me as a science teacher in Monticello Georgia.

# 4

# The Beginning of an Unknown Passion

During the spring of 1994 I scheduled my first out of state interview in Monticello Georgia. Just for the record, the deer population in Monticello far exceeds the human population, as Monticello is named as the deer capital of Georgia. It is also the city where the movie "My Cousin Vinny" was filmed. In the film, actor Joe Pesci played the character as Vinny trying to help his cousin get out of a compromised position. Because they were from New York and visiting in a small town they ran into unfortunate obstacles. In this town everyone knows everybody and when strangers are easily noticed and watched with a close eye. As my brother and I entered on Highway 11 off interstate 20, we became weary of the scenery. There were fewer buildings, cars and people and more grass, trees and farmland. I thought moving from Detroit to Montgomery Alabama was a wakeup call; however, it was nothing like what I was currently witnessing before my eyes. I thought I was driving to the set of the"

Little House on the Prairie". The land and trees were beautiful. Everything looked very peaceful, natural and relaxing. Not a building in site other than a few historic homes with thousands of acres of farmland and organized rows of pecan trees providing shade on the highway. I also had my first experience of seeing and smelling a chicken house

Eric and I were a little nervous visiting such a city as two African American males driving from the Atlanta area. As I went in for the interview, Eric my brother, stayed behind and decided to wait patiently in the car. After the interview I went outside to find a tall older white gentleman about 6"8" standing next to our car. He wanted to know who the person was sitting in the car and what were we doing on campus with an Alabama tag. I immediately made up my mind to not take the job. This guy was one of the most intimidating people I had ever seen. Before I could respond the person finishing up my interview yelled and said, "Hey Mr. Arp, this is Mr. Williams" he is interviewing for the science position for next year". Mr. Arp, said ok, however, he did not relax his face to make a friendly smile, he went on to explain that they were making sure that we didn't have someone on campus with harmful intentions with the Alabama tag. I felt he was cracking a joke, but never got a full smile from him. Instead he reached his hand out to tell me that he was my assistant principal. His hand was three times the size of mine as he firmly shook my hand. I said to myself, there is no way I am taking this job within this town.

Mr. Jordan, then took my brother and I on a tour of the city around the square. The county's population was only 11,000 at the time with approximately 3,000 in the city. A downtown area without a building taller than two floors high within the entire town. A rustic historical looking downtown area with a square in the middle of surrounding small buildings. With a historical courthouse and monument highlighting the view of the square. You can say this was the beginning of a long journey ahead.

The tour was interesting as we visited one of the city diners named Dave's' Barbecue where everyone knew everybody. The food in Dave's smelled like good home cooking. As I walked in, I saw a variety of different people in line for the lunch buffet. Collard greens, corn bread, macaroni and cheese, pork chops, baked chicken, sweet potato pie, mashed potatoes and gravy along with a tall glass of iced tea. You could smell the food before entering the building. I was introduced to several people within the community during lunch. The food was on point, and the hospitality was perfect. You felt like you were with people who knew and cared for you. I guess I could say it felt like home. I knew then that the popular phrase "you can't judge a book by its cover" was true.

That night while watching the NBA playoff game it was interrupted by the infamous O.J. Simpson live police chase. I could not believe what I was watching. We were in a rural part of Georgia unknown to anyone we knew. We were both nervous as hell and immediately locked our doors and did not leave the hotel room again that evening. By the crack of dawn, we were out of there. I remember going back on highway 16 east and hitting the gas until we hit the Alabama line.

I certainly did not think I would ever be going back to this town again. After getting back to Montgomery Alabama, my mom had already received three phone calls as to how they were impressed with me at the interview and how they would love to have me work in Monticello. My brother and I looked at one another and just laughed. Neither one of us expected for me to take the job in Monticello Georgia. What I did not expect was to receive some of the nicest calls after getting back home that I had to take my chances with this new adventure to rural Georgia. My sister had recently moved to Powder Springs GA, so I figured I would not be too far for her in case she needed anything. There were only a few black teachers in the school. Yet I saw the demographics of the student population at about 50/50 black and white. That summer of 1994 I signed my first high school teaching contract for $23,500 a year to teach science in Monticello Georgia. At the time I was the only black academic teacher in the high school or in the district. I said after my first few days this may not be the place for me. I stuck out like a sore thumb.

Yet I met some of the nicest people in the world right in the small town of Monticello Georgia. Mr. Arp the tall assistant principal turned out to be one of the best assistant principals I have ever worked for. He taught me the ropes quick. Always watching for duty and making sure everyone did things on time. He later died after my first three years of colon cancer. I remember him discussing with me some of the treatments and asking me questions about his condition in the teachers work room. After his death, I was shocked as he was the first person close to me to die from cancer.

I worked extremely hard during my first few years focusing on not getting caught up in anything. I remember my first High School principal Mr. Jimmy Jordan, laying it out on the line for us the first day. "Hey this is a small town, you let your hair down everybody is going to know it." Not having much hair, I knew that I was going to make a lot of trips to Atlanta Georgia which was about 45 miles northwest of Monticello. I focused my attention on my career and programs associated with the students.

I will never forget after one of my first staff meetings I meet with one of the veteran science teachers in the building. He said to me with his brown straight hair, and Caucasian colored skin and a foreign middle eastern accent "you're not the only African American in the building, I was born in Egypt you were born in Detroit LOL. We laughed the entire day off that statement. Mr. Eljourbagy along with Jerry Williams, were one of my first mentors in Monticello Georgia. Mr. Eljourbagy recommended that I apply for a position as a science teacher at the Governor's Honors Program of Georgia. I did not think I would get this position as it is designed for some of the most talented students attending schools both public and private across the state of Georgia. Because I was year, teacher from Alabama, I felt surely not to be the first choice. However, when they came to visit my classroom for a few days I began to realize that they were enjoying the topic. I was later informed that I got the position as a science teacher for the Governors Honors Program of Georgia

My plan was to teach for a few years and attend medical school in the state of Georgia. Well that never happened as each year while teaching in my early career I realized that there was something about what I was doing that was uniquely different from anyone else and apparently others noticed a gift I did not see within myself

My first few summers were spent working with the Governors Honors Program of Georgia. After my second year of teaching GHP I interviewed for the Department Chair for the science department and was surprised to get the position. I remember some of my greatest teaching and leadership experiences from GHP. Being a young black male at 26 serving as department chair for science GHP took some people by surprise. I think it took a few people some time getting adjusted, but for the most part I kept it moving. Focusing on the program and the students was my primary goal. The staff became more like family as staying in the same building it seemed as though we grew as friends. Color seemed to be less transparent as I believe our primary goal was to transcend knowledge in the most extraordinary way to the most gifted within our state. The staff and students were always excited to get started and sad when it ended.

I do remember one experience during the summer program in which a group of educators from Germany visited the GHP in Valdosta GA. There was a social event scheduled for all the department chairpersons and the German educators one evening during their visit. As department chair for the science department, I was required and expected to attend this event. As I walked up the stairs of the event several of the German educators immediately looked my way and walked into my direction. I know I was clean but not that clean to get that much attention. The first one smiled and said hello and proceeded to hand me his drink. I did not know what to think as before I could respond I was swarmed with several Germans handing me their drinks smiling nodding their heads as saying thank you. My shirt was wet with spilled drinks. Once my colleagues noticed what was happening, they immediately ran over to inform the Germans that I was the department chair of science. Apparently, they thought I was a butler or waiter because I was a well-dressed young black male attending a social gathering for department chairs of a gifted program in Georgia. They apologized as I threw the cups away, said my goodbyes, and immediately exited the event. I left with a wet shirt, a little disappointment and an opportunity to learn something. They only judged me based on what they were exposed to in Germany. How much history did they know about black males in the United States in 1997? They assumed based on circumstance. Were they to be considered prejudice or un-informed? Did one action from the first approaching person immediately cause the reaction of others. I summed it up, changed shirts and went to local restaurant alone. I did get a surprise as one teacher found out where I was located and surprised me with every one of the GHP staff members from the social event. They all left after hearing the news and wanted to know if I was ok. I was good and was even happier to see all the staff members surprise me. Understanding that racism and stereotypes do exist, and are alive and well, we must remember to not judge everyone based on one person's actions.

During the regular school year most of my time was occupied working with various coaching sponsoring duties. I was both assistant band director and assistant high school basketball coach. Music and sports have always been a natural love of mine. I also served as one of the coaches for the science Olympiad. This left little time for a huge social life during that time. My first three years I focused strictly on my career. Besides the extracurricular duties at school, I also worked as a board member for the Monticello, Jasper County Chamber of Commerce. Eventually becoming the first African American to serve as President of the Monticello Jasper County Chamber of Commerce and serve back to back terms 1999-2000 and 2000-2001.

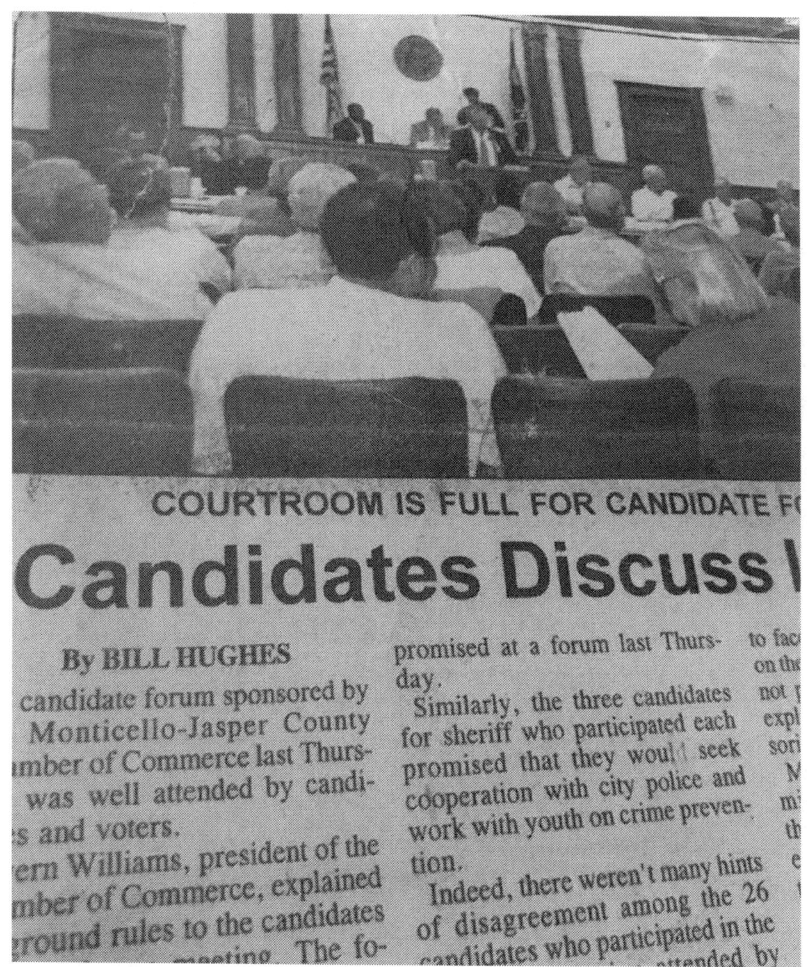

COURTROOM IS FULL FOR CANDIDATE F

# Candidates Discuss

By BILL HUGHES

candidate forum sponsored by Monticello-Jasper County mber of Commerce last Thurs- was well attended by candi- s and voters.

ern Williams, president of the mber of Commerce, explained round rules to the candidates The fo-

promised at a forum last Thursday.

Similarly, the three candidates for sheriff who participated each promised that they would seek cooperation with city police and work with youth on crime prevention.

Indeed, there weren't many hints of disagreement among the 26 candidates who participated in the

# 5

# The Teaching Sauce

Building relationships with students is a primary ingredient for student achievement. As a matter of fact, several researchers do not believe a teacher can truly teach a student unless they build a relationship with them. The question is how do you build a positive relationship with all your students? Do personalities have anything to do with whether one can build a positive relationship or not? A lecture on the epidemic of heart disease, strokes and diabetes brings more of a real-world application to the classroom. Is there someone you know that has survived a heart attack? Or maybe you can discuss the epidemic of kidney failure and strokes. One effective method used in building a relationship with students is to share some of your real-life experiences with the class. Students need to know that you are someone that have overcome obstacles. They may begin to view you as a survivor and respect your opinion as a result of you sharing your experience. This may give educators, students and parents the opportunity to bring forth a meaningful conversation from two different generations on the same topic.

One of the most successful ways of building relationships with students is allowing students to have an open and honest classroom discussion. Students have more questions about the world than we can begin to put into a curriculum unit. Before any discussion I would tell my students to remember to have an open mind. What you know is not what everyone else knows! The way you live is not the way everyone else lives. I normally put the classroom in a circular shape so that everyone is part of one large group. All energy is focused on the center point and no one person is greater than the other. We will then begin our classroom discussions.

I was hired as a science teacher with other duties such as the assistant band director and assistant basketball coach. Monticello had the first flag team in history in 1994. Several of my students have gone on to be successful in their lives and careers. I remember mentoring this one student throughout his high school and college years. I served as his B-Team basketball coach. Odell Thurman will always be that basketball player that goes baseline when we needed a score and somehow always made it. I remember the last year Odell played for me on the B Team. We beat the varsity team and was one game away from going undefeated. On the last game of the year, the head varsity coach took the first- and second-string players from the B Team. We were left with 7 players, all third string. Everyone watched and cheered as the third string players who had little to no playing time had to try to continue to make history by being the only unbeaten basketball team at the school. They cheered the 4th string to a game that ended in a tie as they still ended the season as 13-0-1. We remained undefeated and celebrated not losing a game as if we were winning a state tournament championship. Odell Thurman went on to play for the University of Georgia and was one of the top Middle Linebackers in the Nation. He was drafted in the 2005 NFL by the Cincinnati Bengals. He was nominated as runner up for defensive rookie of the year and lead the Bengal's in tackles as a rookie. Odell's career was short and brief because of an unfortunate epidemic that affects every community. The unfortunate obstacle of substance abuse is a serious issue for all Americans. Although his NFL career was short lived, he will always be considered to me as the best Rookie Middle Line Backer to Play in the NFL.

Coaching as a method of inspiring students has been noted by several researchers as one of the best methods which allows students the ability to reach their full potential. While teaching epidemiology and public health I always try to approach each topic with looking at it from the perspective of the student. I want them to understand that their thoughts and ideas are important to our society. My objective is to serve as a facilitator, coach or guide in the classroom instead of serving as a judge, dictating and dominating every conversation within the four walls. I have learned over the years of teaching that everyone has their own unique teaching style. Unfortunately, all teaching styles are not conducive to learning for all students. Classroom management is another important tool for successful teaching. Some teachers may serve as a judge and jury in the classroom. Directing and controlling every aspect of the classroom. Students must feel free and comfortable to share thoughts.

Motivation is another important valuable characteristic needed for teachers to assist students to achieve academic and life success. Educators must complete several tasks. Beyond the physical task, one must also be reminded of all the other things that students must deal with. Teachers must teach through the mind of a student who may be dealing with the worst of circumstances at that very moment. A great motivator will have the gift of encouraging students through their roughest times. To continue to push the student to reach their absolute full potential is an important part of student success. Being skilled with the idea of knowing when to push and when not to push is the key. If they want to go to the moon encourage them to visit the stars.

Motivation is also used to encourage positive behavior. Students are given gifts for positive behavior as a reinforcement for good behavior. The idea of getting the gift or prize controls the action of those students. What if you can show them how to accomplish their dreams. Will a student become motivated if they felt they had a path to greatness? What if they had someone on their team who really had their back and genuinely cared about their future? I have always tried to motivate and inspire students to move beyond the normal barriers and to understand that no one is like anyone else. We all have different directions that we must take with our different passions.

Amber Broughton never heard of the word epidemiology until she saw it as one of the elective science classes available during her junior year. She took the class and became instantly intrigued by the subject and topics. Amber decided to pursue public health community as one of her gifted an advanced requirement senior project. Amber received her Bachelor of Science in Public health from the University of Georgia in 2016. She received her master's degree in public health in 2018 from Emory University School of Public Health. I am so proud of her for her hard work and accomplishments. I know that her family and friends are so proud of her success. As a gifted student, Amber did not need much to motivate her to pursue her own dreams. She became instantly intrigued by epidemiology and made a career choice as a junior in high school. My role remained as a coach to push her to strive to the highest mountain that she could reach. She currently works in the field of public health.

I have four basic rules I use to motivate student success.

My Ingredient for Motivation.

1. Be your student's biggest cheerleader! Letting all students know that they have a gift for the world. No matter how rich, poor or their cultural background.
2. Teaching students to become resilient in their endeavors and goals.
3. Your life and the life of others is the most valuable gift.
4. Letting them Know you Care about them and their passion.

Recognizing, honoring, and respecting all students is the first step used in letting them know you care about them. Based on my experiences, once students see that you have given everyone a fair and equal opportunity, they tend to begin to believe that you care. Respecting all students regardless of their race, cultural background, gender or way of thinking. Allowing students to open their minds and try to identify their purpose and that they can make the next big change for the greater good of humanity. Teaching them to never quit or give up regardless of their circumstances. No matter what keep pushing forward.

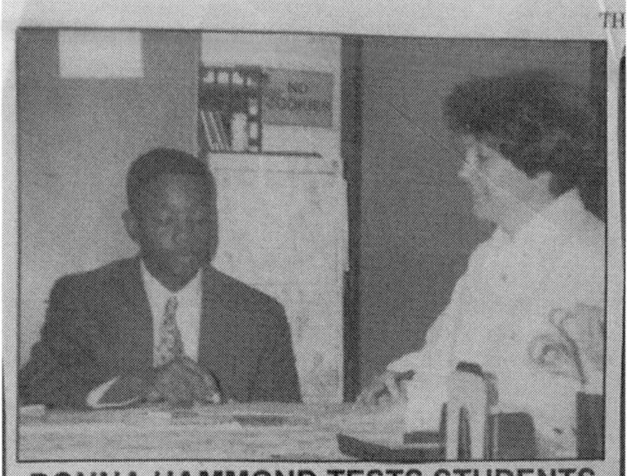

DONNA HAMMOND TESTS STUDENTS

# Local Teachers Offer Input on Testing

By NANCY STAFFORD

Teacher testing in Georgia will be different because of the input of two Jasper County Comprehensive High School teachers.

College graduates who will become teachers will be tested differently beginning in 1997 on the knowledge they should have mastered in their field.

The change in testing brought up the problem of what information future teachers should know and be tested on before receiving a teaching certificate.

Evern Williams, a science teacher at JCCHS, and Donna Hammond, a home economics teacher, were chosen to meet with committees to advise the testing service on solutions to these con-

The Educational Testing Services asked college professors and secondary teachers to form panels to look at specific areas of concentration.

Each panel was made up of 12 members from diverse backgrounds that were considered very knowledgeable by the testing service.

"The meetings were filled with discussions and sometimes heated debate on issues such as relevant and irrelevant content, the cut of the scores for passing, whether the test should be essay or multiple choice, and if the test should be comprehensive or should be broken into specific sub fields," according to Mr. Williams.

"One of the biggest problems was trying to create a test that would

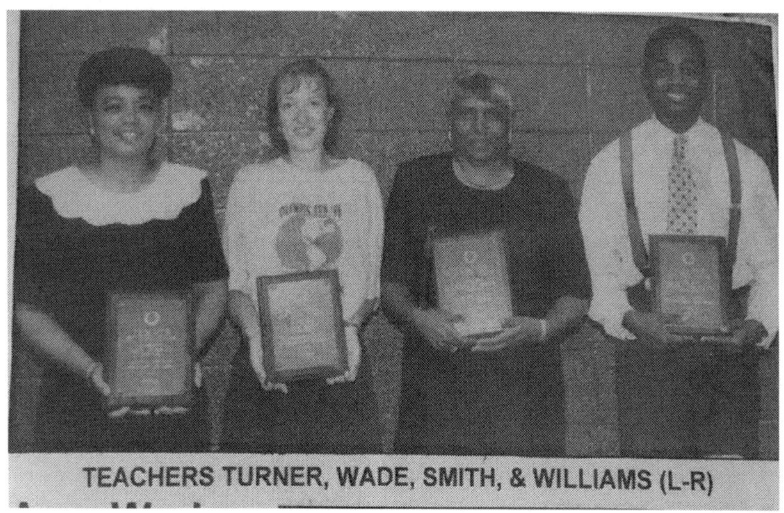

TEACHERS TURNER, WADE, SMITH, & WILLIAMS (L-R)

Teaching them to think outside of the box is an important component of teaching as it prepares them to learn from others around them. Everything that you believe may not necessarily be correct. You may soon realize that some of your beliefs regarding health and life is merely a myth supported by irrelevant, non-researched information passed on from different people within the environment.

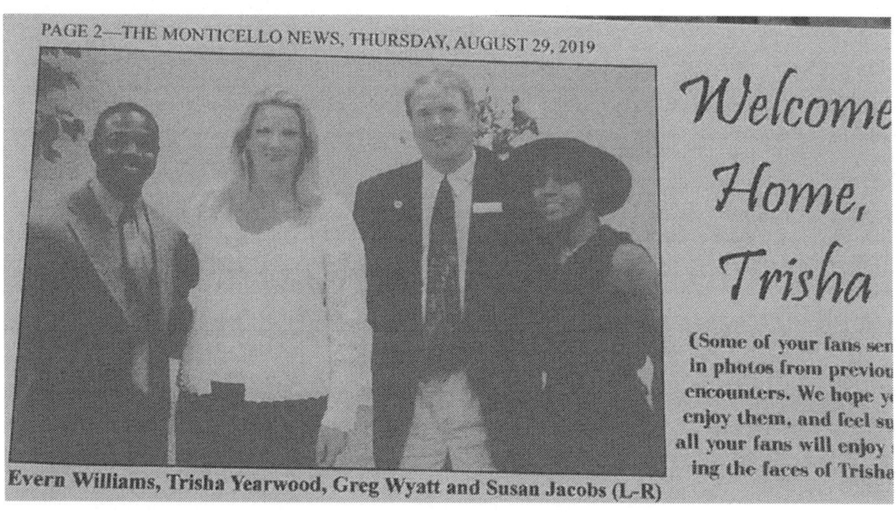

PAGE 2—THE MONTICELLO NEWS, THURSDAY, AUGUST 29, 2019

Welcome Home, Trisha

(Some of your fans sen in photos from previou encounters. We hope y enjoy them, and feel su all your fans will enjoy ing the faces of Trisha

Evern Williams, Trisha Yearwood, Greg Wyatt and Susan Jacobs (L-R)

I believe in working hard both in the community and in the school building As, a former coach, I always found myself as a mentor advisor to hundreds of students. In 2010 I ran into one of my former students who had recently won the My Black is Beautiful contest and was featured on the cover of the Essence Magazine. She later won the title of Ms. Georgia and won 2nd Runner up for the 2013 Ms. America Contest, Ms. Tiana Griggs. It has always been the greatest reward to see some of those you have worked with or taught in a successful career or pathway. Jaylinn Mann, one of my students who hated science entering the 9th grade yet is currently a medical school student at Morehouse School of Medicine.

A third important tool needed is to nurture or groom students. Some students need to be guided to their destiny. Coaching and motivation may not be enough. These students need those who can nurture and groom them to success. I describe these moments that your students need you to take on the role of a personal advisor. Documents for college, forms for a scholarship as well as to continue to push them to join various organizations that may assist in building experience in a specific field or career choice.

What are the characteristics do I have that motivates them based on their opinion? The only way of getting this information is to ask the students. So, I decided to ask my students in my last epidemiology classes from 2017- 2018. What are the characteristics I demonstrate most that encourages you to learn? The students discussed these characteristics in my presence openly and explained each in detail, I took notes. The characteristics are in no specific order although the first 7 were named first by most of the classroom.

1. Allow students to share information without judging them.
    a. *Students may have interest that may get your attention or something you may have in common*
2. Do not be ashamed to share downfalls or unfortunate experiences with the students.
    a. *Students need to know you have overcome obstacles*
3. Do not portray that your perfect or that you have no weaknesses

    *"We all have something we need to work on"*
4. Become Culturally sound and have an open mindset for discussion
5. Give students meaningful work instead of busy work. Real world application of knowledge as opposed to basic standardized test.
6. Allow students the opportunity to not be perfect or have a plan, allow them to develop their own passion without passing judgement.
7. Maintain a supportive and professional relationship with students.
8. Understanding distinctive characteristics of all students and respecting those characteristics.
9. Maintain some form of flexibility and encouragement for student work and achievement.
10. Allow students the ability to challenge or question procedures democratic practices in the classroom.

11. Never lose a student's trust.

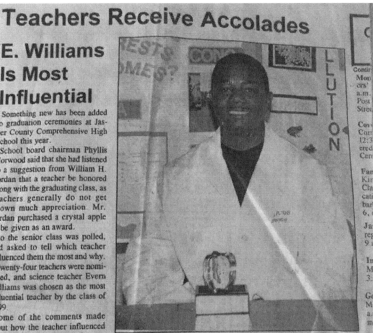

# Teachers Receive Accolades

## E. Williams Is Most Influential

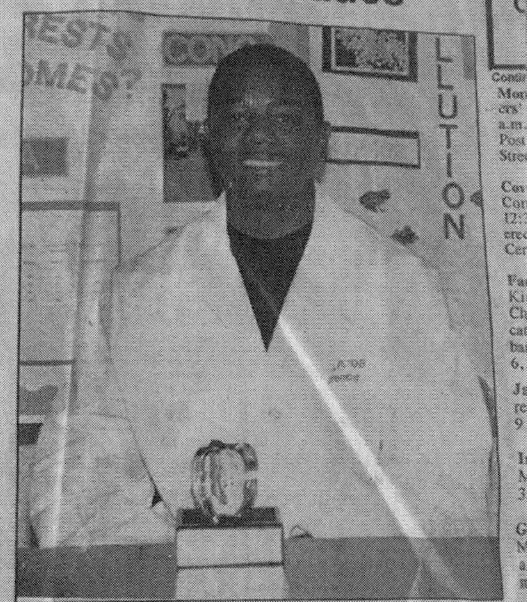

EVERN WILLIAMS WITH CRYSTAL APPLE

Something new has been added to graduation ceremonies at Jasper County Comprehensive High School this year.

School board chairman Phyllis Norwood said that she had listened to a suggestion from William H. Jordan that a teacher be honored along with the graduating class, as teachers generally do not get shown much appreciation. Mr. Jordan purchased a crystal apple to be given as an award.

So the senior class was polled, and asked to tell which teacher influenced them the most and why.

Twenty-four teachers were nominated, and science teacher Evern Williams was chosen as the most influential teacher by the class of 1999.

Some of the comments made about how the teacher influenced the students' lives included:

Mr. Williams "was real; straight from the heart," "He is very inspirational...he always stresses the importance of education," "Mr. Williams gets to know his students as an individual, not only as a class that he has to come in and teach. He is very dedicated, honest and trustworthy to his students."

Also, Mr. Williams "always keeps it real." "He encourages students to learn because it's fun, and not because of test or quizzes. He has told me that I can be anything and he's pushed me to work for everything I desire. He is so intelligent and truly a wonderful human being."

Several other teachers were also

something out of myself." "She motivated from the beginning to the end of the year."

Mrs. Sara Hayes—"Mrs. Hayes has really inspired my life...she always helped me to achieve any goal sought. She always encouraged me. She told me, 'No matter how tough it gets just hold on, keep the faith, and all of your dreams will come true. She is truly like a second mother."

Mrs. Nona Arp—"She brought excitement to the classroom that made science and math interesting and fun. Also, not only is she a great teacher, but she would be a friend to her students."

Mrs. Lois Turner—"When I was

me to try my best and to excel at my school work." "He influenced me more than words can say." "He helped me prepare for the hard work that was ahead of me."

Mrs. Janice Moore—"She has taught me how to believe in myself and she has taught me how to think positive." "She helped me with all my problems in my life. She helped me with my reading and school work." "She's always there to work with someone and help with anything, even things she does not teach."

Mrs. Amy Cheek David—"She has helped me with my graduation test, and she is a good and caring teacher."

Mrs. Dianne Irwin—"She has pushed me to do so many things

When you are working in a small town it does not take long for the word to get around. If your horrible everyone will know it and if your gifted, they will recognize it as well. After working with several people within the community your name begins to get around as Mr.

Williams can fix it. I had one young man approach me as I was a part owner of a store with his father. Meathead, at the time now known as Future, asked me to be his manager when he was a teenager. I told him I would love to help him, but I was no manager for the music industry. I promoted concerts in my earlier days with the Goodie Mob, of the Dungeon Family. As he shared some of his thoughts and ideas, I remember thinking that this is one smart young businessman, always seeking more knowledge and always ready to learn. Another group of young men I had the opportunity to work with were the Levitt brothers in Covington Georgia. They are two that avoided the gang world by building the foundation of the Gentlemen's Club in Newton County. From a life that could have gone to gangs to a life of both graduating and living successful lives in the military and the music industry. The guys are also talented musicians, which was an immediate connection which transcended to one of the largest male organizations on campus. Stepping and providing community service the young men formed a fraternity of love that led hundreds of young men on campus into the right direction.

Unfortunately, there are so many students who did not have the same outcome. After teaching for more than 25 years I experienced losing hundreds of students due to various epidemics within our community. Car accidents, homicide, kidney failure, suicide, and opioid addiction. The more I began getting into the topics in class, I knew that this was a class that all students could benefit from regardless of color, race, spiritual belief, or gender. I always followed the motto of treating every student as if they were related to me in some way. Students need to know that you care about their future. Influencing students to reach their greatest goals is and has always been my motto. I would always tell my students, “regardless of your current circumstances you can control your future by securing it with your actions today

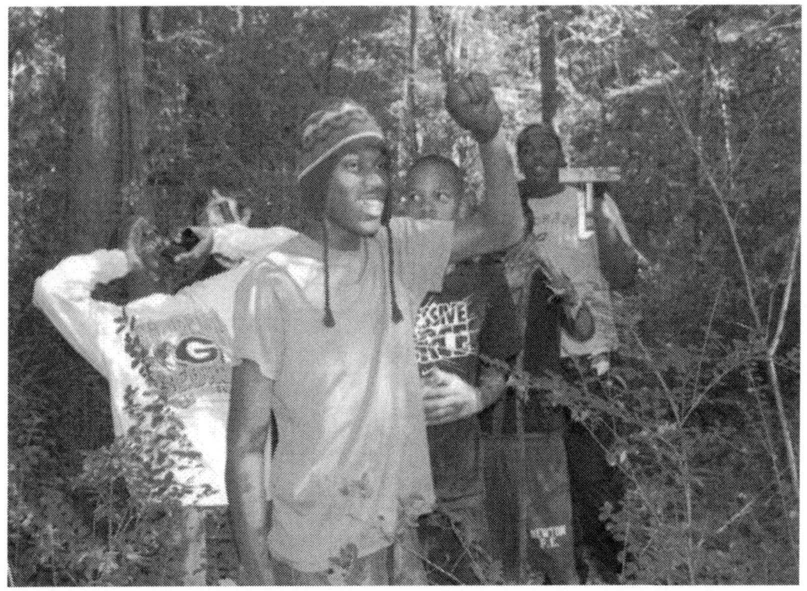

Students working on community service project 21st Century After School Program, Newton High School 2012

# 6

# The CDC Discovery

With all the opportunities emerging within the field of education, I decided to explore this career and the options within it. For the next three years I decided to be the best science teacher I could possibly become. What I did not realize was that becoming a successful teacher required one to meet several goals that may seem to be unrealistic. I vowed to be different and learned how to embrace my uniquely different qualities to enhance the educational experience for our children.

The average curriculum included math, science, history, English, physical education, music and the arts. This was before STEM, a familiar acronym describing science technology engineering and math. School systems continued to offer the same standard classes maintaining the identity of each discipline taught without including integrated curriculum. There were no advanced placement classes or gifted programs in several districts. There was no such thing as gifted endorsement for teachers either.

During the summer of 1996 I began my new position as the Science Department Chair for the Governors Honors Program
of Georgia.

# Mr. Williams Redesigns Curriculum

Evern Williams, teacher and chairman of the science department at Jasper County Comprehensive High School, hass been asked to redesign the curriculum for the science department of the Governor's Honors program (GHP).

The request came from the state department of education which administers GHP.

The new curriculum, which will be written by Mr. Williams, will offer new ideas and innovative strategies to provide the honor students with a more successful GHP experience.

Last fall, Mr. Williams presented his curriculum plans to the state department, and the state curriculum coordinator and the director of GHP reviewed and accepted the plans.

The new curriculum will emphasize group research which gives [illegible] rience since most science research projects are done primarily by groups. The curriculum will also include interrelated seminars in which the students will see how each area of science relates to one another as well as how each area has a significant important in every day life.

The curriculum will be put into action with this year's GHP program which begins this month.

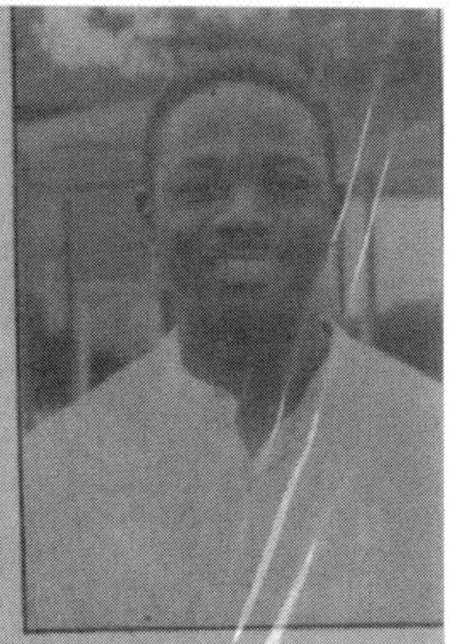

EVERN WILLIAMS

Article from Monticello News.

I finally had the opportunity to teach about the HIV epidemic during the summer in the GHP. Thinking that this would be a class that was relevant, as HIV was then known as the deadliest sexual transmitted disease within the United States. Discussing this topic could possibly save the life of a student or someone they love. The following year the CDC approached the Governors Honors Program of Georgia with the idea of teaching TEAMS and acronym for Teaching Epidemiology to All Middle School Students. They wanted to offer a trial run with the students and faculty from the science department of the Governors Honors Program of Georgia. The information was to me certainly more suitable for high school students than middle school students. The students were given a real-life case study from a true outbreak of legionnaire's disease in Bogalusa Louisiana. They had to navigate through the outbreak to find out the source of the disease. The objective was to get them to think as a disease detective researching and trying to find out the cause of a problem based on detailed information from the outbreak. During their journey, they will learn the principals of epidemiology and public health. We unpackaged the information and disseminated different areas to the students with the CDC monitoring and evaluating the case study. After the lesson, the science staff meet with officials from the CDC to discuss the pros and cons of the pilot. I suggested that the information and curriculum was more suitable for high school students and everyone agreed. I saw the various compartments within the curriculum that would truly make for an exciting integrated curriculum including other subject areas. The CDC seemed interested in what I was describing in the meeting and agreed to allow me to show them how to integrate the curriculum back at my high school in Monticello, Georgia. I noticed how all the different subject areas could teach possible teach the same topic from different perspectives related to their subject area. Math worked with data analysis including, interpreting data, odds ratios, probability, and forming charts and graphs. Biology focused on the bacteria the physiology, morphology and lifecycle of the legionnaire's bacteria. While the band learned the theme song 007. Since it was not common for the CDC to visit a high school, a local news crew from channel 46 came to film the project and interview us afterwards. After the visit, the CDC decided to get me more involved into the project.

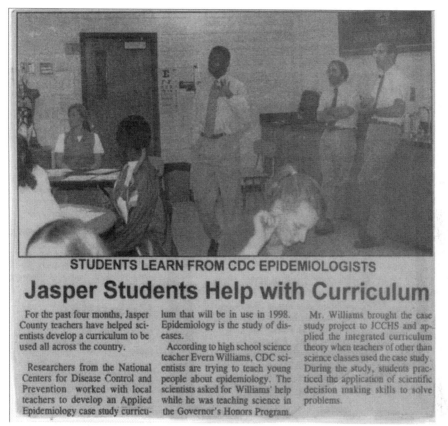

STUDENTS LEARN FROM CDC EPIDEMIOLOGISTS

## Jasper Students Help with Curriculum

For the past four months, Jasper County teachers have helped scientists develop a curriculum to be used all across the country.

Researchers from the National Centers for Disease Control and Prevention worked with local teachers to develop an Applied Epidemiology case study curriculum that will be in use in 1998. Epidemiology is the study of diseases.

According to high school science teacher Evern Williams, CDC scientists are trying to teach young people about epidemiology. The scientists asked for Williams' help while he was teaching science in the Governor's Honors Program.

Mr. Williams brought the case study project to JCCHS and applied the integrated curriculum theory when teachers of other than science classes used the case study. During the study, students practiced the application of scientific decision making skills to solve problems.

Monticello News

After the visit, the CDC decided to name the teaching module, EXCITE, an acronym for Excellence in Curriculum Integration through Teaching Epidemiology. I was pleasantly surprised and thankful to receive a contract in 1996 by the CDC as a consultant for my expertise in teaching the principals of epidemiology to teachers. I was hired to serve as a consultant to the EPO department under the guidance of Dr. Stephen B Thacker.

**Picture of faxed Contract!**

AH06M224 SUPPLIES SERVICES 12/11/2000
REQUISITION-NO: EPO103-01 INQUIRE MODE PAGE: 1

| ITEM-NO | SUPPLIES/SERVICES | QUANT. | TOTAL | OBJ | CAN CODE |
|---|---|---|---|---|---|
| 1 | CDC REQUESTS THE EXPERTISE OF MR. EVERN WILLIAMS AS PART OF CDC'S EXCITE PROGRAM (EXCELLENCE IN CURRICULUM INTEGRATION THROUGH TEACHING EPIDEMIOLOGY). MR WILLIAMS AS CHAIR OF THE SCIENCE DEPT. OF THE GA GOVERNORS HONORS PROG. WAS INSTRUMENTAL IN ADOPTING EPIDEMIOLOGY IN SCIENCE TEACHING IN 1966. SINCE THAT TIME HE HAS HAD SIGNIFICANT EXPERIENCE USING EPIDEMIOLOGY AS A CURRICULUM IN INTEGRATED TEACHING. HIS SERVICES AS A CONSULTANT ARE NECESSARY TO ADVISE CDC ON HOW TO DELIVER CURRICULUM MATERIALS TO TEACHERS. | | | ---- | -------- |

( -- )ENTER NUMBER OR USE PFKEY FOR DESIRED OPTION
1: COMMENTS 2: LAST SCREEN 3: PREV PGE 4: NXT PGE 5: SEL PAGE 10: MAIN MENU

EXCITE, an acronym for Excellence in Curriculum Integrating through Teaching epidemiology served as a module for teachers across the nation. From the EXCITE Curriculum module emerged several entities such as, Disease Detectives, Science Olympiad, and Science Ambassadors Program for teachers.

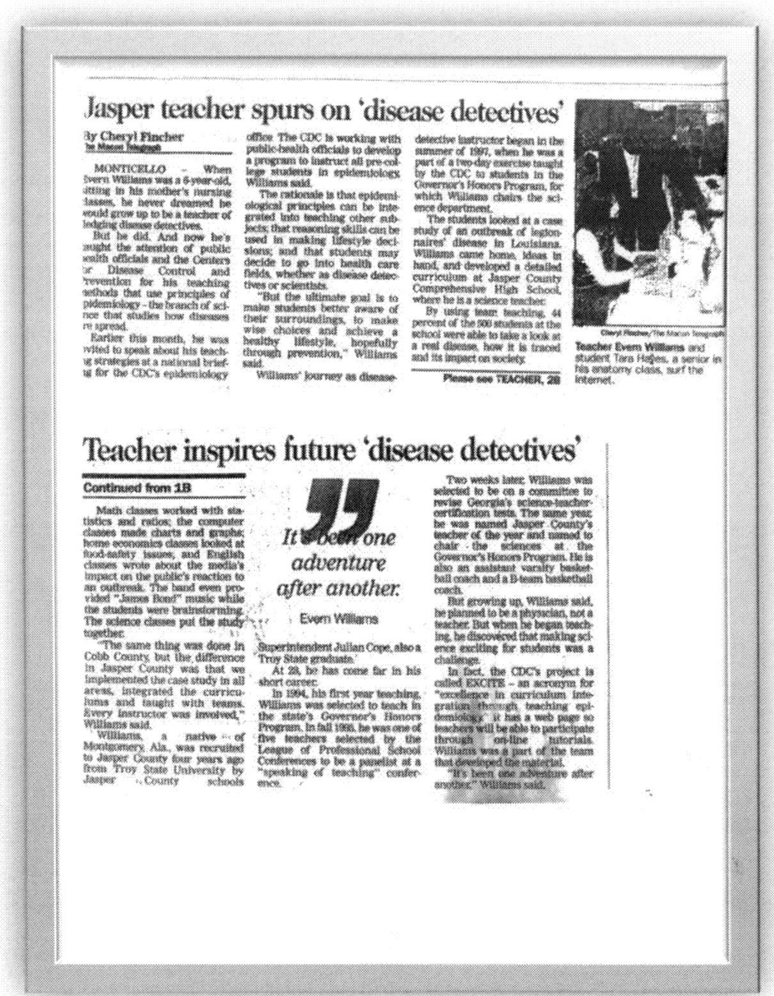

## Jasper teacher spurs on 'disease detectives'

By Cheryl Fincher
The Macon Telegraph

MONTICELLO – When Evern Williams was a 6-year-old, sitting in his mother's nursing classes, he never dreamed he would grow up to be a teacher of fledgling disease detectives.

But he did. And now he's caught the attention of public health officials and the Centers for Disease Control and Prevention for his teaching methods that use principles of epidemiology – the branch of science that studies how diseases are spread.

Earlier this month, he was invited to speak about his teaching strategies at a national briefing for the CDC's epidemiology office. The CDC is working with public-health officials to develop a program to instruct all pre-college students in epidemiology, Williams said.

The rationale is that epidemiological principles can be integrated into teaching other subjects; that reasoning skills can be used in making lifestyle decisions; and that students may decide to go into health care fields, whether as disease detectives or scientists.

"But the ultimate goal is to make students better aware of their surroundings, to make wise choices and achieve a healthy lifestyle, hopefully through prevention," Williams said.

Williams' journey as disease-detective instructor began in the summer of 1997, when he was a part of a two-day exercise taught by the CDC to students in the Governor's Honors Program, for which Williams chairs the science department.

The students looked at a case study of an outbreak of legionnaires' disease in Louisiana. Williams came home, ideas in hand, and developed a detailed curriculum at Jasper County Comprehensive High School, where he is a science teacher.

By using team teaching, 44 percent of the 500 students at the school were able to take a look at a real disease, how it is traced and its impact on society.

Please see TEACHER, 2B

Cheryl Fincher/The Macon Telegraph

**Teacher Evern Williams** and student Tara Hayes, a senior in his anatomy class, surf the internet.

## Teacher inspires future 'disease detectives'

Continued from 1B

Math classes worked with statistics and ratios; the computer classes made charts and graphs; home economics classes looked at food-safety issues, and English classes wrote about the media's impact on the public's reaction to an outbreak. The band even provided "James Bond" music while the students were brainstorming. The science classes put the study together.

"The same thing was done in Cobb County, but the difference in Jasper County was that we implemented the case study in all areas, integrated the curriculums and taught with teams. Every instructor was involved," Williams said.

Williams, a native of Montgomery, Ala., was recruited to Jasper County four years ago from Troy State University by Jasper County schools Superintendent Julian Cope, also a Troy State graduate.

> It's been one adventure after another.
>
> Evern Williams

At 28, he has come far in his short career.

In 1994, his first year teaching, Williams was selected to teach in the state's Governor's Honors Program. In fall 1996, he was one of five teachers selected by the League of Professional School Conferences to be a panelist at a "speaking of teaching" conference.

Two weeks later, Williams was selected to be on a committee to revise Georgia's science-teacher-certification tests. The same year, he was named Jasper County's teacher of the year and named to chair the sciences at the Governor's Honors Program. He is also an assistant varsity basketball coach and a B-team basketball coach.

But growing up, Williams said, he planned to be a physician, not a teacher. But when he began teaching, he discovered that making science exciting for students was a challenge.

In fact, the CDC's project is called EXCITE – an acronym for "excellence in curriculum integration through teaching epidemiology." It has a web page so teachers will be able to participate through on-line tutorials. Williams was a part of the team that developed the material.

"It's been one adventure after another," Williams said.

Monticello News

For Twenty years EXCITE served as the premier educational tool for teachers provided by the Centers for Disease Control and Prevention. After EXCITE, the CDC began developing other programs such as the Science Olympiad competition curriculum and Science Ambassadors. Science Ambassadors was a program developed to train teachers how to come in and write a curriculum with CDC experts. These teachers are selected from a pool of applicants nationally. They are invited to live in Atlanta and train for a week with public health scientist, statisticians, and medical doctors. After the one-week training with CDC staff members, the teachers are to present their lesson plan to the public health and educational community. The lesson plans were placed on the CDC's website for teachers to utilize as a tool for teachers in the classroom.

From 1997 to 2001 I traveled with the CDC during the summer months and weekends as an expert consultant in teaching the principals of epidemiology in high schools. Presentations included the following schools and or venues, Princeton University, Woodrow Wilson Institute, University of Georgia, Emory University, The Centers for Disease Control and Prevention Center, CDC, National League of professional Schools Conference in Bellevue Washington and The State Science and Technology Conferences in Georgia. A CDC official and I was even invited to discuss the project on one of the most popular radio stations in the south, V-103.3 Frank-Ski and Wanda's Morning Radio Show.

# Mr. Williams Speaks on Atlanta Radio

Jasper County High School science educator, Evern Williams, recently made a live radio debut on the WVEE 103.3 morning show in Atlanta speaking about the Center's for Disease Control (CDC) EXCITE project.

The EXCITE project was piloted by Mr. Williams at the Governor's Honors program in Valdosta during the summer of 1997 while he was chairman of the science department. The project was later implemented at Jasper County High School. It is now being used across the country by several high schools, colleges and universities.

Mr. Williams was joined on air by Dr. Donna Stroup, CDC official, who informed listeners of the teacher's web page for the project.

"It was something very different for me; speaking without seeing my audience. You can imagine my excitement when the radio producer phoned to schedule the interview," said Mr. Williams.

# Mr. Williams Teaches at Princeton

Evern Williams, a local science teacher at Jasper County High School traveled to Princeton University in Princeton, NJ this summer to participate in a two day seminar with officials from the Centers for Disease Control (CDC) in Atlanta.

Last year the CDC and Mr. Williams began working on a curriculum designed to teach students the principles of epidemiology (the study of diseases) by using the scientific method. The CDC originally had planned to implement it in middle school science courses only.

Mr. Williams expanded on this idea and designed a plan to integrate the entire curriculum in several different subjects--math, computer science, biology, family and consumer science, health occupations, and special education. Thus, a collaboration was born.

These classes were all involved, simultaneously, in the case study be implemented at Jasper County High School and the Governor's Honor Program. After visiting the school, the CDC named the project *EXCITE: Excellence in Curriculum Integration through Teaching Epidemiology*.

Last spring Mr. Williams attended a CDC meeting with Dr. Bob Moore, State Science Curriculum Coordinator, and some of the CDC's leading epidemiologists to discuss methods of promoting this project to the nation.

The Woodrow Wilson Foundation

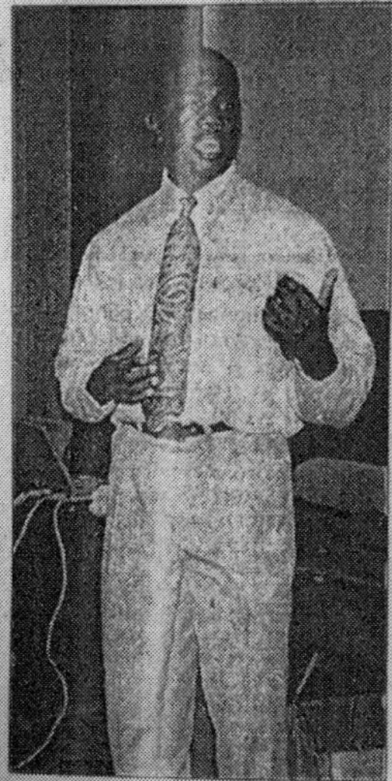

EVERN WILLIAMS

Mr. Williams also had an opportunity to meet Richard Preston the author of the book *THE HOT ZONE*. This book is about a true outbreak of the Ebola virus. Mr. Preston discussed with Mr. Williams his involvement with the CDC and the ideas of integrating the curriculum to teach outbreak principles.

Mr. William's presentation was attended by Mr. Preston, who is

Since Princeton there have been invitations to present the project at several conferences across the country.

"I've been invited back to Princeton next summer and I am looking forward to the experience," says Mr. Williams. "I am very excited about *EXCITE* and the positive impact it is having on our school system and Jasper County."

"I credit Jasper County with a very large part of the projects' success nationally, as well as my own. It all started here and be assured my immediate future plans are to continue teaching here in Jasper County."

The CDC will host an EXCITE workshop October 2 and 3 in which Mr. Williams will be presenting.

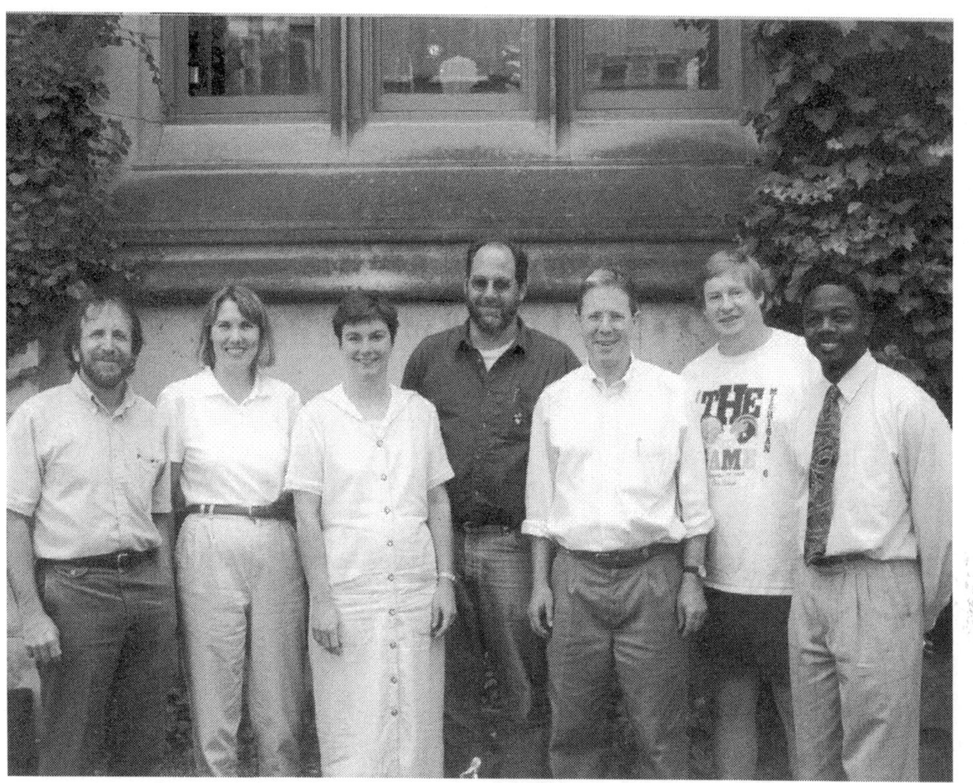

Rick Goodman, Ruth Berkelmen, Donna Stroup, Andrew Goldenkrantz, Richard Preston, Evern Williams; This picture was taken after the Presentation for the Woodrow Wilson Institute for Teachers at Princeton University 1998.

While visiting Princeton University with the CDC, I was fortunate to have the opportunity to meet Richard Preston, author of the book, "The Hot Zone". Richard Preston and I had some great conversations at the dinner table. We shared some of our personal hypothesis of phenomena within the United States. We were both like kids in a candy store sharing and bouncing ideas off one another.

Our conversations were interesting enough for Richard to decide to attend our presentation scheduled for the next morning at Princeton University where he surprised the audience by giving an impromptu discussion at the end of our presentation. I remember our discussions which led to the idea of offering a student handbook for his novel, "The Hot Zone". "The Hot Zone Student Handbook" was written by Andrew Goldenkranz one of the coordinators of the program and Richard Preston. I highly recommend "The Hot Zone" by Richard Preston as a reading in any public health and epidemiology class. This book shows the devastation one virus may have on humanity and works great for classroom discussions and scenarios related to a real disease threat.

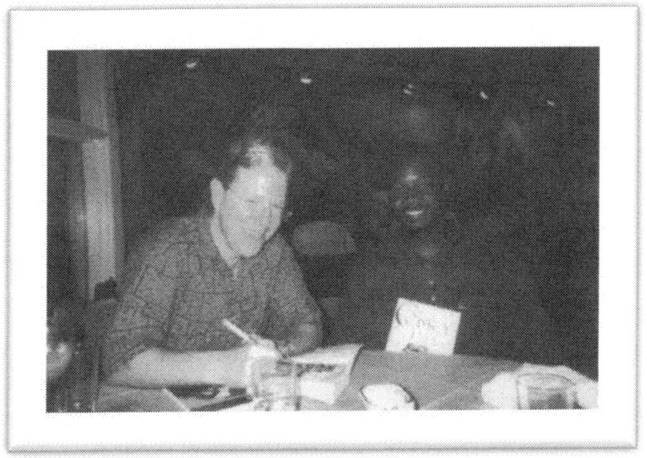

My path in life has afforded me the opportunity to work with a remarkable organization and some of the brightest men and women within the public health profession as well as directly work with students and parents from rural and urban areas. I was also afforded the opportunity to travel a path and endure a journey that has afforded me the opportunity to touch lives. Whether the topic is discussed inside or outside of a classroom, learning and understanding how these frameworks work may serve as a helpful tool in teaching students how to problem solve. If we learn how to analyze and determine cause and effects of problems, then we may learn how to apply this knowledge to help resolve our own problems.

7

# The Evolution of Public Health

Most people do not know the history or purpose of the Centers for Disease Control and Prevention Center. Several people associate the CDC with infectious disease prevention and research. The CDC was established in 1947 as an organization designed to study research and prevent the spread of malaria. The name of the CDC was called Communicable Disease Center, with Dr. Joseph Mountain serving as the director of the organization in its earlier days. The CDC is funded by the federal Government and serves as the leader in public health for the World Health Organization and global public health awareness.

When it comes to public health, disease, safety or anything that may cause harm to an individual the CDC is keeping up with the statistics of these problems. Maintaining proper data and monitoring these trends for changes in numbers is the way in which the CDC surveillance public health.

When is it ok to discuss suicide, one of the fastest growing epidemics with intentional self-harm (suicide) reporting more than 47,000 deaths a year in 2017 in the United States? https://www.cdc.gov/nchs/fastats/deaths.htm. Or the number of homicides of black males within the community? Currently, community epidemics are on every television channel, and or social media outlet. These epidemics not only affect student decisions but their futures as well. I believe public and private educational services can provide a valuable vessel to teach all students how to live a safer and healthier lifestyle by offering epidemiology and public health classes. For more than 22 years I have had the opportunity to teach thousands of students, staff and health professionals the principles of epidemiology and public health. Students have shown great interest as several have pursued careers in epidemiology and public health. Others have developed life skills that has afforded them the opportunity to reach their full potential. My motto has always been "Keeping it Real". That is not only the motto that I live by but also the motto that I have learned to teach. Epidemiology is real. In fact, it is about as real as a problem that you can properly identify based on statistics.

Alcoholism, drug addiction, poverty, and mental illness all play an important part in the overall academic achievement of students. How can we encourage students who face these various challenges without discussing the specific problems within their communities?

If you ask yourself right now what the ten biggest problems children, teenagers and young adults struggle with today will likely be on the list of community epidemics. These epidemics are largely responsible for the deaths of various subgroups of individuals including all ages from infants, to the elderly. The word epidemiology is the study and analysis of cause, effects, and patterns of health, disease and social action that may affect a specific population. For most adults, the word epidemiology is a word that is rarely heard by friends or family yet is however more commonly mentioned on the news. Coronavirus, HIV, Homicide, gang violence, poverty, media influence, addiction, human trafficking, car accidents, suicide and Ebola are all epidemics recently experienced by our society. With such a wide variety of topics covered under the epidemiology umbrella one must ask the question, "What is the common characteristic? How can we integrate or teach such a wide variety of topics in one class? How can we provide this information for students within a curriculum already bound by guidelines and policies that may restrict teachers from new subjects that are not proven to be research based? Considering all the various components of teaching a diverse class, I focused on the common denominator. The common denominator involved math as all epidemics are determined based on numbers interpreting trends.

For years scholars have pursued the idea of making math relevant, yet when teaching science, math takes a preferential front seat to other subjects. Epidemics are based on data results. When the numbers exceed normal rates or statistics it may be recognized or considered an epidemic. The study of epidemiology and public health allows students to understand why a specific problem may be considered a health risk and what can be done to reduce those risk. Pandemics are epidemics that have spread globally allowing students the opportunity to gain knowledge from a global perspective. To understand epidemiology, one must have a basic understanding of cause and effect. What are the causes of the problem and what effect does it have on the population? Furthermore, the effects of some human behaviors may cause or encourage an outbreak. Epidemics are researched so that scientist and public health officials can analyze, detect and try to reduce a specific problem or disease from spreading. Currently there are more than 790, 000 heart attacks in America each year. The CDC indicates that someone in America is having a heart attack every 40 seconds. For the most part, when there is an increase in frequency, or how often it occurs, it may be considered an epidemic.

Heart disease has always been an epidemic increasing in cases every year. The average adult knows someone who may have died from a sudden heart attack with no previous signs or symptoms. Epidemiologist study problems affecting a population as opposed to a medical doctor who studies the health of a specific individual. In the case of heart attacks, epidemiologist would diagnose, analyze, and study how to prevent the number of people dying from heart disease each year, while developing and implementing prevention methods based on research. What are the different causes of heart attacks? What is the history of heart disease in America? Are their behavior risk factors that may increase the chances of someone having a heart attack? What is the best way to disseminate information on health risk to the community? Teaching students about public health provides relevant information that will help students make better decisions regarding safety and health. When we speak of problem-based learning we must consider current problems within our communities. Students may be more likely to gain interest in a topic that they have experienced. Epidemiology leaves no one out! Everyone has experienced losing someone to a specific epidemic. Therefore, everyone has a common denominator in an epidemiology classroom which is relevant and based on real world topics and health concerns.

How do we teach students to solve real world problems? Would it make any difference if these problems were relevant to them or not? Teaching students how to live a safer and healthier lifestyle is not only relevant but necessary. If we want to teach students to become problem solvers, we must put them in a position to solve a problem. Students can study a variety of topics while researching problematic factors such as global socioeconomics, religion, politics, statistics and literature. What is the cause of the problem and what are the long and short-term effects of this problem on the individual and their community? In some cases, or epidemics, the effects of someone's actions may allow him or her to increase their chances of becoming a statistic. Ethics must be considered as several laws and policies may not only reduce an epidemic but aid in increasing those numbers.

There are several different categories of epidemics. Infectious disease, geriatrics, chronic disease, social, behavioral, and occupational epidemics. The various categories cover a large area of health threats to the community. Students are also given the opportunity to study the various public health careers.

Coronavirus is one of the latest epidemics that serves as a threat to the world. The coronavirus began as a threat in China during the later month of January 2020 and within one month the virus has made its way to every continent across the globe. According to the CDC and the World Health Organization, the Coronavirus has similar characteristics of the common influenza Virus. They both cause fever, chills, coughing, sneezing and shortness of breath. Since both are viruses a vaccine is the only medicine that can be given to an individual to prevent them from catching it. At the current time there is no vaccine available for the coronavirus. There were similar viruses such as the Hong Kong Flu which killed more than 1 million people worldwide in 1970. Fifty years later a new Corona Virus has become one of the most talked about topics around the world. When teaching students about the coronavirus I first began with the history of this virus from both the distant past and recent outbreak. I also remind students to focus on where they receive information as several media outlets may utilize this outbreak as an opportunity to spread misinformation for personal profit. Descriptive epidemiology identifies the person, place and time of the victims of this outbreak. This enables the students to see the detailed characteristics of those infected and dying from this disease. All people are susceptible of catching this disease, however several of the victims dying from this disease seems to be older senior citizens and younger children. At the current time more than 700,000 people are known to be infected with the Coronavirus in the United States and more than 80,000 people in China. According to reports, more 55,000 deaths have resulted in the United States while only 3500 deaths in China. I emphasize how analytics plays a role in describing the impact of such an outbreak. Comparing the number of deaths caused by the influenza virus which was responsible for more than 60,000 in 2018 and the deaths in the United States due to the Coronavirus which may exceed 60,000 deaths alone. There is a vaccine for the influenza virus which can prevent someone from catching this bug, but there is nothing prepared for the coronavirus that may spread without a known vaccine. This is what may be considered one of the most challenging ways to contain the coronavirus. Ethics will discuss procedures for containing the virus which includes quarantines and screening to identify those who are infected. Also, the economic devastation it may have on our society including travel, cruises, and large entertainment venues may have less in attendance because of the threat. New rules for various cities now requiring all those in public to wear a mask and practice social distancing. Public Health surveillance will continue to monitor the number of new cases and continue to inform the public of current relevant information needed to reduce the spread of the Virus. The same efforts and strategies to prevent the spread of influenza are the same for the coronavirus. Making sure you thoroughly wash your hands, wearing a mask, keeping a safe distance from others , enforcing the stay at home if your sick policy for all employees and to clean and disinfect door handles and other items that people may publicly touch. This is a current and true outbreak which is a great way to discuss all the teaching methods that will more likely get several to change behavior patterns that may help reduce the spread of the infection.

As I began my quest, I never imagined in my lifetime that something this devastating would emerge. Unfortunately, we all have endured the burden of modifying our lives for something non-living, that we cannot even see. And since a virus is a threat that we cannot see visually with the naked eye, most people may not believe that it exists. We must understand that all forms of life and non-life may pose a serious threat to humanity. Based on the history of viruses in the United States alone allows one to see how viruses have impacted our society in the past. Students, parents, counselors, teachers and citizens should benefit from learning how to protect their families and their communities.

# 8

# Epidemiology on The Move

When I hear that our students in the US ranks far behind other countries in math and science I began wondering why. Our students constantly struggle with science, math and reading. As an adult we tend to read things that are of interest to us. I would like to believe students would read more if they were provided more interesting things to read. Epidemiology provides topics and case studies that may directly affect any population. Infectious disease outbreaks from both past and present such as Coronavirus, Bubonic Plague, smallpox, HIV, and Ebola are discussed and studied in an epidemiology classroom. When describing the symptoms of someone infected with the Ebola virus, every student was on the edge of their seats. Some immediately asked the question, could we possibly catch something like that? It was at that point that I realized they wanted to read more about the virus themselves. Several came back to school the next day describing things they read on their own without it being assigned as homework. They were interested in something that may affect them.

First High School To offer Epidemiology to High School Students:

The very first state to offer Epidemiology in public schools was Georgia. Newton High School was the first public high school to offer Epidemiology as a science course during the 2011-2012 school year. Students enjoyed the class and was fascinated by the amount of relevance and real-world problems that were investigated and studied. The class was originally thought to be a course for the gifted and was quickly changed to include all students. The idea was to provide all students the opportunity to learn public health. The class offers teenagers the opportunity to identify a variety of health care careers and local health care facilities. A sense of excitement was always in the air as they knew they would learn something new each day. My first topic was on the epidemic of HIV in America. It gave them a unique perspective on how everything within a system affects an epidemic.

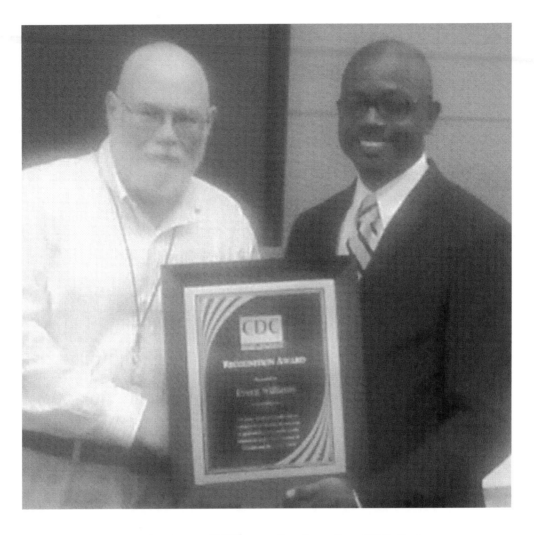


**Ralph Cordell, Evern Williams During the CDC Science Ambassadors Ceremony 2011**

**Evern Williams Receives Pioneer Award by the CDC for his Leadership in promoting the teaching of public health and Epidemiology to Students in Georgia and the United States**

After teaching Epidemiology for the first year it became the most popular selected elective class for the year of 2012. At this time there were restrictions placed on the requirements for the class in order to equally distribute all the other science classes. Various groups of students loved the class, from special needs to gifted students, they all were excited to take Epidemiology. From the very first class in 2011 more than 70 % of that class went on to pursue careers in public health.

**Local Newspaper Students Comments.**

Not only do the students get a top-notch teacher, they are also the first public school class in not only the state, but the nation, to be taught the subject of epidemiology.

If the name does not ring a bell do not feel bad. Most of the students had no idea what the class was even about when they first heard of it. But it caught junior Amber Broughton's attention immediately.

Amber Broughton, “I did my homework," she said with a giggle. "But the name interested me immediately."

Epidemiology is the study of the causes, distribution and control of diseases in populations. But more than that, it shows how a disease can effect a community - such as the student population at NHS. The course also looks at how anything may affect a population, such as teen pregnancy, car accidents and even homicides.

"I didn't expect it to be how it is," said junior Jeremy Laguins. "It's like real stuff, real facts that I never knew, and I never really thought about... It's straight from the CDC and I really like that."

From AIDS to rabies, the students are being challenged not only to think and learn, but also to discuss and debate numbers that all questioned agreed they found shocking.

"The first week we took samples around the school and put them on auger plates," said Broughton. "Just seeing how filthy the most common areas you touch every day are. Oh my God."

All the students now always carry hand sanitizer around with them.

Jeffery Fallah' “It's really hands-on and I am a hands-on learner,". "...It's something new every day. I feel like I'm being taught by a college professor."

For senior Sarah Knight, the epidemiology class helps her with her goals of entering the medical field.

Sara Knight Senior, “I feel like this helps me get my foot in the door," she said. "...We sit in the classroom and have a debate and he's on our level. He is not talking down to us. In fact, he's told us a few times that he's astonished of what we think and how we think."

https://www.covnews.com/news/education/cdc-teacher-a-pioneer-in-epidemiology/

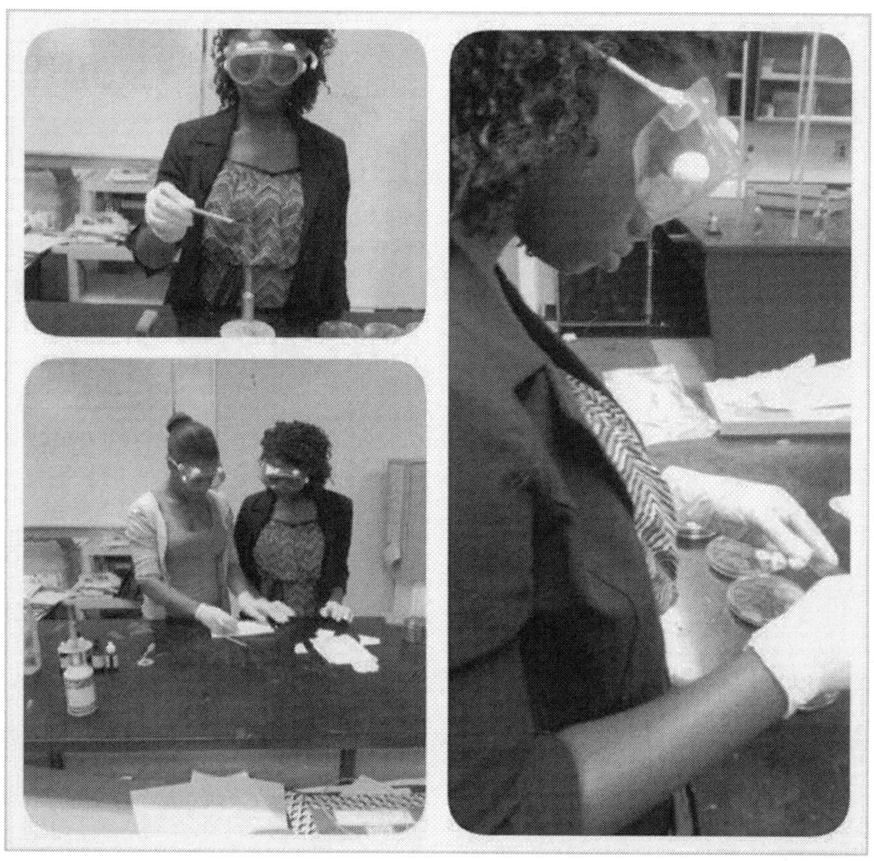

Several others have gone on to work within a variety of health care fields and pursue public health degrees. This course also allows students the ability to study and understand how culture and social norms may affect scenarios.

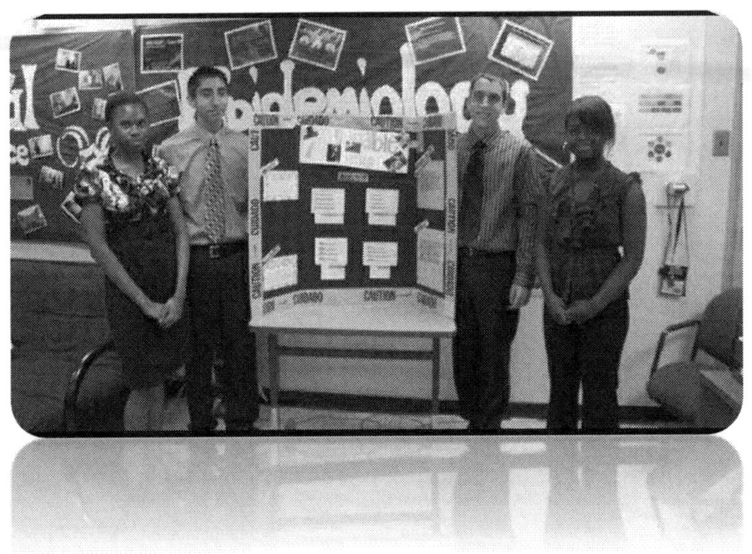

Students learn how everything within their immediate surroundings may affect their outcome within an epidemic. It teaches students the importance of data and how to rely on it as well as research-based methods and theories.

After 2011 I felt destined to continue my quest for pushing epidemiology in all schools. I was the guest speaker for the next two graduation ceremonies for the Science Ambassadors program held at the CDC during the summer months for teachers. With the change in leadership my work with all projects including speaking at the graduation ceremony for the CDC ended. The framework I began working on developed into the Core Competencies for High School epidemiology and public health which is currently on the CDC's website.

I remember reaching out to several of the states resource departments for teachers and asking to teach teachers and administrators the principles of epidemiology and public health, and being informed that this is not the type of science or subject area that's relevant enough at the time. STEM and robotics were the primary objectives of science teachers. I remember thinking that epidemiology is a STEM class. As a matter of fact, it was a STEM class before STEM existed in my mind. And how many robotic tools are used in modern science and health. I realized that if not needed now then one day it will be necessary for all to understand and learn the principles of epidemiology and public health. I knew the topic and class was unfamiliar to most, so I was very understanding as to why several were not too excited to train for such a class. I remembered watching Oprah Winfrey discuss the topic of "Purpose" with one of her guests which really put things in perspective for me. I began to understand my purpose and why I continue to move on a path different than others. Your purpose is your purpose, and it is for you. We always wonder why certain things happen to us both good and bad but at the end it is all about your purpose in life.

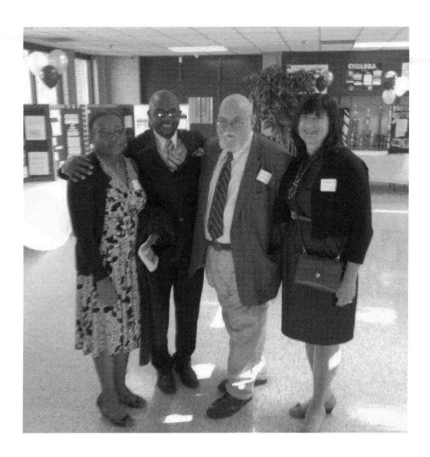

Dr. Ralph Cordell, Esther Shisoka, Karen Seals and Evern Williams

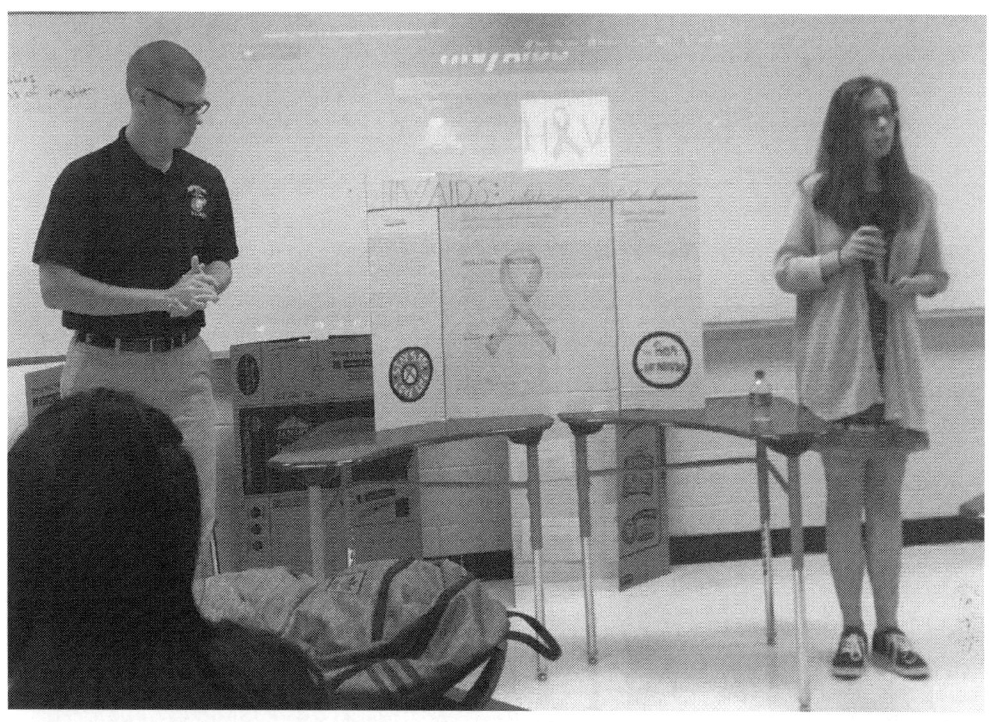


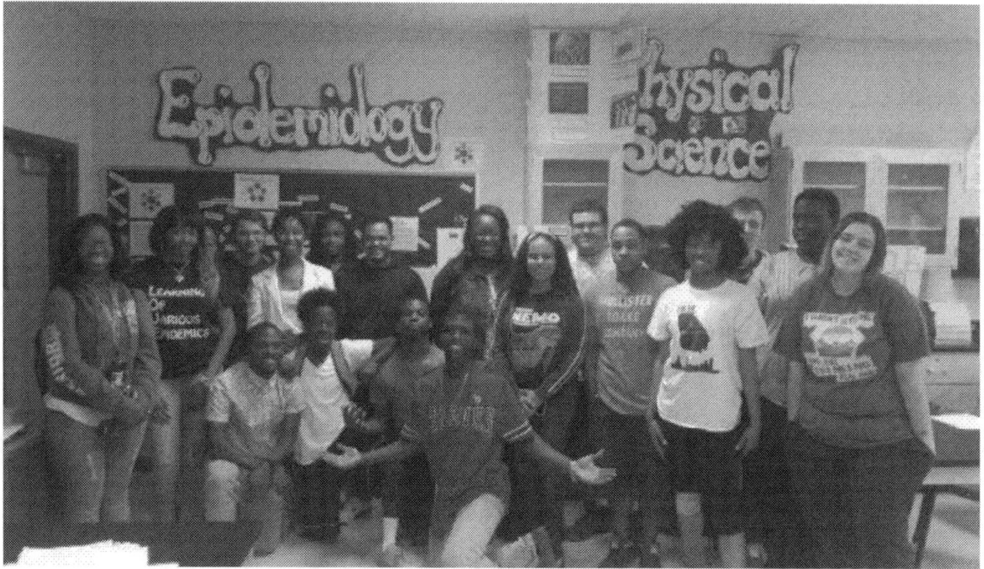


Over the past 9 years I have presented at both state STEM and Georgia Science Teachers Association Conference. Introducing the concept of teaching high school epidemiology and public health.

Although most was not sure what to expect, more than 90% of those attending my presentations always gave positive reviews. Teachers and administrators may also develop skills by learning epidemiology. Teachers have become inspired to teach classes and offer more topics over the years.

Teachers Participating in an Epidemiology Activity Georgia State STEM Conference

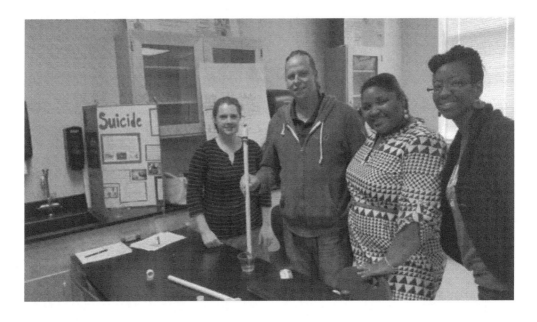


District Level Professional Development Newton County Schools 2015

Most educational institutions mission statements include providing students the academic skills to become successful academically and socially. We want students to be lifelong learners and to develop problem solving skills that may assist them with solving problems amongst their peers. Over the past 400 years education has essentially been the same. The technology has advanced over the years to assist us with the task of teaching, yet what we teach and how we teach has continued to remain the same. How do we teach problem solving skills without discussing daily problems?

My experience has revealed to me that this class and the methods used were immensely helpful in building respect for all cultures? Could teaching epidemiology and public health to all students give students an opportunity to learn of the various pitfalls they may face within their own environment? Or can teachers gain an understanding of cultures by teaching epidemiology? Can we teach the epidemic of poverty, drug addiction, homicide, suicide and human trafficking as a public health problem in schools? Discussing topics such as these may provide an outlet for students to open about personal issues within their lives. The questions are endless. Yet our student's future and success are merely a reflection or measurement of our work. Teaching a student how to problem solve is teaching them how to design a map through some of the toughest obstacles they may have to face in their lives. No, it is not the answer to every problem it just gives them an opportunity to better prepare for and avoid obstacles.

# 9
# Five Frameworks

After the FLU EXIT Project with the CDC, I received a request from Georgia Department of Education by way of the CDC to assist in designing some sort of framework for teaching the epidemiology in high schools. I scheduled a meeting by phone with Mr. Juan Carlos at the time who served as the state curriculum coordinator from the Georgia Department of Education. After the meeting I began designing a framework to teach epidemiology to high school students. I began to think as a student. What would make epidemiology in public schools interesting and enjoyable for students? I did not want to lose the students interest and stay within the guidelines of the Georgia Science Standards and Next Generation Science standards. Epidemiology covers several different topics. Almost anything can become an epidemic so where do you begin as an educator. I first imagined myself as a high school student sitting in a science classroom viewing all the different topics of epidemiology. How do I get my students to think like an epidemiologist? How can I get them to become problem solvers? The first thing I thought of was how to disseminate the information in a way that will allow them to understand the information without confusion. I compared the knowledge students receive and learn to a deep freezer. As educators we sometimes give information to students in lecture form without providing a conceptual framework. What is a conceptual framework? Conceptual framework is an analytical tool used to identify different variations of information. It is used to make conceptual distinctions and organize ideas as it relates to a specific topic. I needed to take the public health and epidemiology umbrella and compartmentalize the major areas of study, so that our students will begin to think like an epidemiologist. What caused the epidemic or what is the effect of the epidemic are important questions. Categorizing the information so that every student could understand and distinguish different ideas of the topic. Like a refrigerator compared to a box freezer. The freezer is not compartmentalized therefore it may be more difficult to retrieve specific items without the frustration of moving items around to find it. In a refrigerator, most of the items are compartmentalized in different categories. Fruits and vegetables, sandwich meats, and milk are all located in a specific location which makes it a lot more convenient to find what you want.

The five Conceptual frameworks selected are described as History, Descriptive, Analytical, Ethical and Public Health Surveillance. I have also come to terms that the five frameworks serve as a primary tool for problem solving. With the wide variety of topics and subjects within the public health curricula, the frameworks provide an essential way to categorize the information received. This framework allows one to organize the information and understand the relevance of each category within it. A nice module that can be used to teach the community how to problem solve.

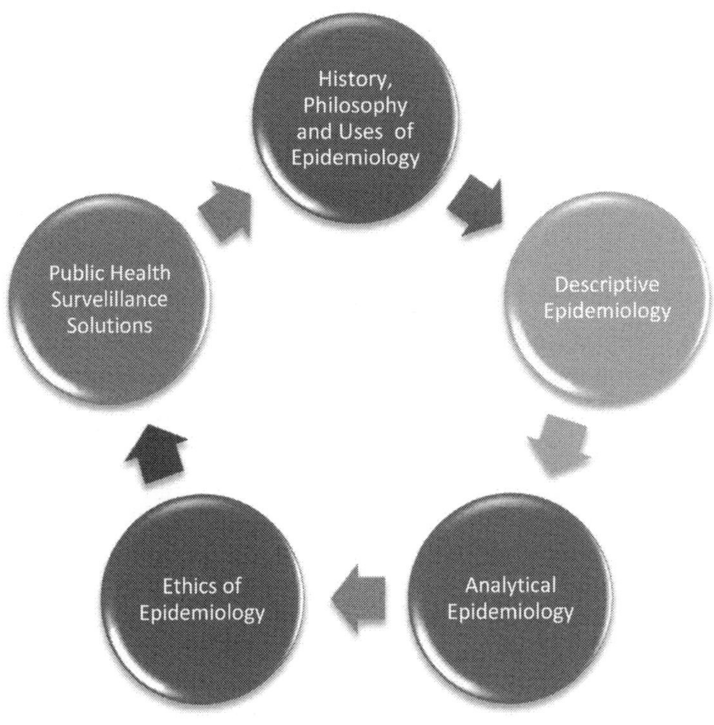


History generally gives the background information of a specific epidemic. The year in which it occurred, how it normally affects the body as well as cause and effects. History also describes the human immunological response to an epidemic. How has the human body responded to viruses? The second is Descriptive Epidemiology which indicates person, place and time. Who is affected by this epidemic? What is the geographical location of the outbreak and when did the public health problem occur? Third is Analytical Epidemiology. Analytical epidemiology framework which involves understanding trends using data. Analyzing the data and researching the problem requires students to understand how to use mathematics when understanding and solving problems. You observe the math and begin to use that math to understand trends. Analytical Epidemiology can become as broad as the student and instructor may want to go. A math instructor may engage the student into the level of math that may meet the individual students learning level. Students can learn how to view, read, understand and interpret charts and graphs, inverse ratios, statistics, case control and cohort studies. The fourth framework is Ethics of Epidemiology which to me is a combination of religion, politics, laws, culture and social values. What may be legal to some may not be ethical or legal to others. This is based on various values within our current society, which includes social, justice, equal rights, culture, laws and policies. Can some policies and laws influence an epidemic? What are HIPPA Laws and why was it so important during the time of the HIV outbreak? Public Health Surveillance and Solutions is the fifth conceptual framework as it is based on observations of programs, dissemination of information and implementing new ideas and or solutions in order to reduce public health risk. It is also based on making observations of the current policies, solutions, programs and determining whether they are reducing the epidemic.

For example, during the year 2005 the CDC launched a massive campaign to remove cigarette smoking from public facilities in the Atlanta area. This was supported by the evidence of their studies done that describe the effects of secondhand smoke. In this scenario students may see how policies and laws may affect an epidemic. Recently the President of the United States restricted travel from Europe to reduce the spread of the Coronavirus here in the United States on March 11, 2020. Policy plays an important role in the containment and to reduce the spread of an epidemic.

The study of epidemiology and public health relies heavily on the team efforts of various public health professionals. Students may explore the various public health careers and understand how these professionals work as a team in solving real-world problems.

**History and Philosophy of Epidemiology**

When anyone of us begin to solve a problem, we must first study the history and characteristics of the problem. History describes the basic history of a public health problem. The data both historical and current determines whether a problem will be considered an epidemic.

This unit provides students with an opportunity to develop an understanding of the history of epidemiology and the various methods epidemiologists use to describe the frequency, course and risk factors for infectious diseases. History of a disease or outbreak may include the following: Past outbreaks, Symptoms of disease, treatment, geographical location, dates, and data or statistics.

The history of how an outbreak affected a community or country is especially important when examining the source of the problem. Not only does this strategy work for epidemiology classes but most project presentations throughout the curriculum would benefit from using a basic framework for project based learning and nonlinguistic representation of knowledge.

The history of a specific disease and or health risk will be reviewed as students will need to understand and gain background knowledge of an epidemic before researching the health problem. Characteristics of pathogens including anatomy, physiology, lifecycle and its historical effects on the human population will need to be included in this section. In addition, students will need to know the body's natural immune system response to infections. This is important to know as it is crucial to understand mutations and morphology as an important aspect of a disease outbreak. Applying scientific research knowledge will enable students the opportunity to experience real-world problem-solving skills. Students will learn how to organize and prepare research results for presentations using history as a primary framework for preparation.

In all subjects and or topics, history has always been an important part of the learning process. Imagine discussing a topic on any subject without your teacher or professor mentioning anything about the history of the topic. History gives you general information regarding a topic as well as the time to research past similar outbreaks. Smallpox was one of the first major viruses eradicated over the last 100 years. It answers the simple question where we were then and now. Is smallpox still an epidemic? Why or why not. For any epidemic, history is useful information as it lays down the foundation of knowledge. The history of the flu virus in America has changed with advancements of science with innovative vaccines and other useful preventive information provided. With the current

Coronavirus outbreak, we may find it important to understand the early stages of similar past viral pandemics.

One would need to know the works of Dr. John Snow and his contributions to public health. Dr. John Snow is considered the father of epidemiology by public health educators across the world. Dr. John Snow investigated one of the first known cholera outbreaks during the year 1854 in London England. Dr. Snow created and used what is called the first spot map ever in diagnosing an outbreak. He is considered the pioneer of epidemiology.

Dr. John Snow identifies clusters of cholera cases in London England by creating the very first spot map

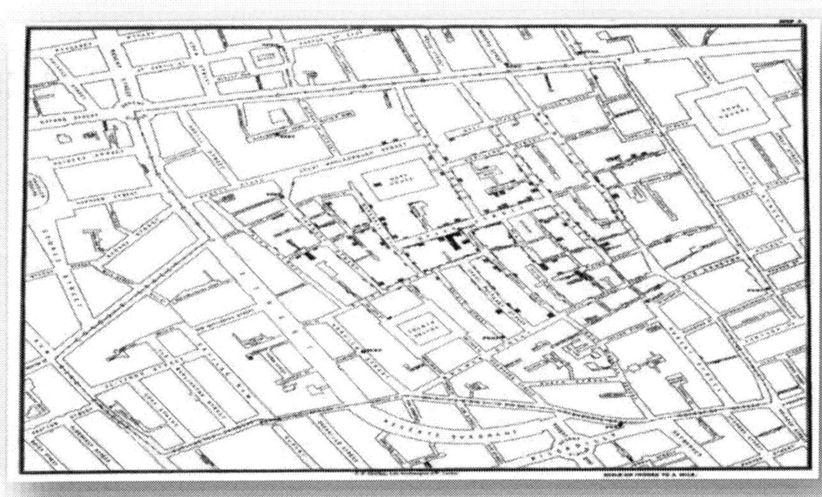

https://www.google.com/search?rlz=1C1CHBD_enUS800US800&q=Dr.+John+Snow+pioneer+spot+map&tbm=isch&source=univ&sa=X&ved=2ahUKEwj61IX0usXoAhWvnOAKHbohBDQQsAR6BAgJEAE&biw=1366&bih=695#imgrc=8pdWxvFrp3jzQM

When teaching my students about HIV, or AIDS, Acquired Immune Deficiency syndrome. Learning the history of this disease has led to several questions regarding its origin and the advancement in science and social equality. As an 11-year-old child I can remember the year 1981 when Prince Charles married, princess Diana and when "We Are the World "was one of the most popular songs in the world. The song was a fundraiser for famine relief in Africa. Another popular discussion of history revealed that GRIDS was the very first name given to the common HIV or AIDS epidemic. Almost all the first known HIV cases were homosexual men between the age of 25 to 45 years of age from New York and San Francisco. There were no known cases of this disease affecting heterosexuals until years later which led scientist and public health officials to change the name from GRIDS to AIDS.

For every topic discussed in epidemiology, the disease detective would need to know the history of a specific scene or epidemic. From Ebola to car accidents, history and philosophy would need to be a vital part of the concept for learning public health.

Mark Kaelin from Montclair State University and I meet in 1997 at Princeton University, he went on and developed the 12 Enduring Epidemiological Understandings. It outlines major objectives students should learn after finishing a unit or activity from epidemiology. The twelve enduring understandings also align with the problem-solving framework.

## Framework 2) Descriptive

Descriptive is a term used in public health which gives details to history. It gives clarification to person, place and time. While researching public health risk, knowing person, place and time is important. However, it is especially important in the understanding and learning of all subject areas. Who, where and when did a certain event occur is a quite common question asked in several subjects? Categorizing information into the descriptive category allows students to easily recognize key components of resourceful information. The Enduring Understandings of Epidemiology describes descriptive epidemiology as a vital resource in its understanding of public health research. When solving any problem, we must identify person, place and time. It also allows students the opportunity to study various cultures, religions, and political views.

Everyone may remember the Ebola outbreak of 2014 beginning in Northwest Africa. It was an epidemic because the numbers of cases far exceeded normal numbers. Person is important because it identifies all those infected. It describes all the characteristics of those infected including, gender, age, race, culture and religion. Place and time are also important in understanding location and time in which an outbreak has occurred. Western Africans were becoming contaminated with the Ebola virus within their communities during the months of June 2014 thru November 2014. From this information, a student can begin to study the different variables that may affect the likelihood of infection. Causation is described as the reason or initiator of a specific situation or event. What may be some of the causes of the 2014 Ebola epidemic? The location of an outbreak may be a determinant factor in the likelihood for contracting a disease. The time of the outbreak, during the summer and fall of 2014 is also important. Person, place and time, is essential for understanding any outbreak or public health threat. As students begin to learn how to investigate an outbreak, he or she will begin to record accurate numerical data as it relates to the outbreak. This is how both descriptive and analytical epidemiology fuse as both are needed to show true cause and effect.

One of the most valuable tools I have learned to utilize in the classrooms is free to the public, yet full of resourceful information for students learning of the various current epidemics at real time. This website www.healthmap.org. links the public to up to date outbreaks anywhere around the world at current time. It is very resourceful and beneficial in educating and teaching young adults' outbreaks within cities and counties next door that may pose a public health risk.

**Framework 3 Analytical**

Analytical is described as analysis of characteristics, and numerical data references. Information on types of study designs, statistical analysis, mathematical computations and research methods used to study public health threats. Analytical epidemiology allows students to categorize numerical data, understand types of study designs, interpret data and how to use this data to investigate prevention effectiveness. Within this framework is where students can focus on the mathematical aspect of epidemiology which measures causation, study designs, odds risk and prevalence. Analysis of data including percentages, graphs and statistical interpretation are discussed. For each case study important statistical data and numerical information is relevant and needed in order to develop solutions. The common denominator for every epidemic is that the number of cases has increased. This unit provides students with the information to understand the research methods involved in Analytical Epidemiology. Analytical epidemiology differs from descriptive epidemiology in that it explains how and why an epidemic occurs as opposed to person, place and time. The students will learn the basic study designs used to determine factors that influence the rate of disease. They will understand how behavioral, biological, demographic and environmental influences affect the rate of a disease outbreak. They will also learn how to implement the scientific method in both an experimental and observational study design. Epidemiological studies look closely at the statistical relationship between factors and diseases which enables students to see whether a certain factor is associated with or causes a disease. The students will also learn how to perform several research studies such as cohort, case control, and cross-sectional studies. Learning analytical epidemiology will give students a real-world application of utilizing critical thinking skills and scientific research methods in order to make decisions which may save lives and prevent the spread of infectious diseases.

What is the one thing that all epidemics have in common? Most people will find this challenging to answer because some epidemics are caused by pathogens while others are caused by social behavior and or policies. Mathematics and data determine whether something is an epidemic. One great characteristic of Epidemiology and public health is that all the topics are real world problems. These problems are proven by data and statistical analysis. Students can understand the role mathematics play in the fight against public health threats.

For any public health issue to become an epidemic, the numbers must be greater than normal. In 1982 there were many people complaining of pneumocystis pneumonia. This increased number of people diagnosed with pneumocystis pneumonia would be considered an epidemic. Epidemiologists investigate these epidemics with the objective of preventing, the spread of it throughout the population. Mathematics is always relevant while teaching epidemiology. As I mentioned earlier, students and teachers can go as far as they want to go with the math. They have the option to explore several different levels of mathematics for a variety of learners. From basic charts and graphs to statistical analysis, public health offers a wide variety of math and how it is used in the real world. While teaching epidemiology in a high school it is good to use a variety of resources for your class. Public Health is one of the fastest growing professions in the U.S. since 2011.

One of my favorite resources I use in teaching analytical concepts of public health to students is Active Epi. Active Epi was written by David Kleinbaum. A good friend of mine who happens to be one of the most popular epidemiology textbook writers in the world.

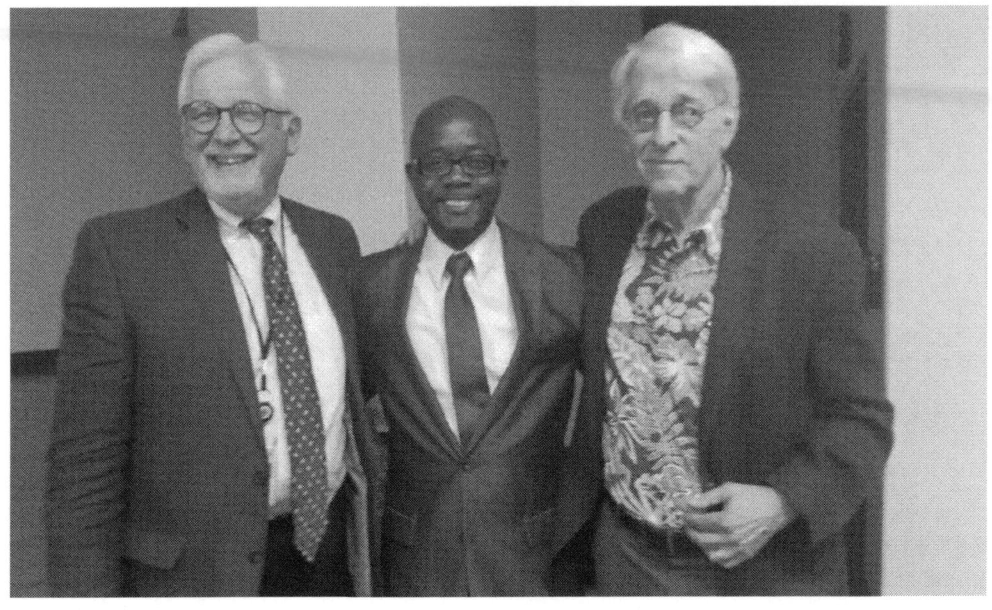

Mr. Dennis Bega, Evern Williams, and David Kleinbaum after a Student led Symposium on Epidemiology and Education Newton College and Career Academy 2015

David has written and developed a product that is useful in teaching students' analytical epidemiology. Active Epi shows students how math is used to identify trends in epidemiology. The book is full of lessons on epidemiological study designs, including case studies, odds and risk ratios and stratified statistics. It allows students the opportunity to see how math is used to diagnose and show trends in data. These activities provide students with opportunities to experience a wide variety of lessons. This is a resourceful tool to use while teaching public health as it provides students with a real-world experience of the analytics of epidemiology. David Kleinbaum is a retired Emory professor of Epidemiology and Public Health. He is probably the most well-known authors of epidemiology and public health textbooks in the world, writing and publishing more than 12 public health and epidemiology college textbooks. Kleinbaum later saw the need to provide public health to high school students. He designed Active Epi years ago and recently upgraded the book to a digital program that is now available to everyone for free. Active Epi has virtual lessons which provides a variety of experimental designs mathematical formulas used for public health research.

I have used this book as a resourceful tool in teaching the Analytical Framework of epidemiology. What does it mean when you hear the word odds ratio? Most people begin to get a headache thinking about the math involved with public health which can be a challenge if you are not mathematically inclined. How would one determine the odds? What does it mean when someone says a boxer is favored to win with the odds at 42:1? I used sports because that is where we feel most comfortable discussing odds and ratios either in sports or gambling. The odds of winning the Powerball. One of the activities in Active Epi written by David Kleinbaum, describes the odds of one getting lung cancer from smoking cigarettes.

In one of the Lessons of Active Epi Kleinbaum describes how to determine the risk ratio of smokers who have had heart attacks will survive by quitting smoking. First, I could not believe they could get people for such a study, yet they found 156 people who had a heart attack and smoked. A much larger surprise was that out of the 156 heart attack smokers, 75 (group A) continued to smoke after their heart attack while the other 81 (group B) stopped smoking. The patients were monitored for five years to see the number of people dying from each group. After 5 years the number of people dying from the stop smoking group (B) with 81 stop smokers was 14 compared to group A with 75 nonstop smokers reporting 27 deaths. Kleinbaum shows students how to perform a simple risk ratio.

Step 1. Students will perform a percentage to get a ratio.

Group (A) continued smokers: 27/75 = 0.36 deaths.
Group (B) smokers who quit: 14/75 = 0.17

This mathematical equation can be interpreted by stating, 36 % of group A died compared to 17 % of group B. The ratio below showing the estimated risk as two to one or shown as 2:1.

$$\text{Estimated Risk Ratio:} = \frac{\text{Estimated Risk for Group A}}{\text{Estimated Risk for Group B}} = \frac{.36}{.17} \quad 2.1$$

Ratio of 2:1 or two to one.

This was one of the first cohort studies done under the American cancer society in the early 1950s. Active Epi has more than 15 chapters which covers a broad range of mathematical curricula from graph interpretation, experimental study designs to statistics. Here we see how math becomes a language and describes a trend. A trend represented and supported by real data and true statistics. Kleinbaums' contributions to education and public health continues to be a vital resource for the field of public health and epidemiology.

## Framework 4 Ethics

Ethics is based on politics, religion, culture and the law. This category is important because it provides the parameters of any experiment, case study and or policy. Students will have the opportunity to relate classroom problem solving and understand why and how policies and laws are implemented. The Red Cross never required HIV testing for donated blood until after they realized the infection was transferable by blood contact as well. I am sure some remember when a bloody nose or jersey was common to witness during a sporting event. A football or basketball game could end up with bloody jerseys worn throughout the game. After the AIDS epidemic, policies and laws were made to prevent the spread of the HIV infection. These policies and laws transcended down to sporting organizations as well as all professionals requiring direct contact with people. Certain trainings were established to prepare all public heath employees to prevent the spread of the infection.

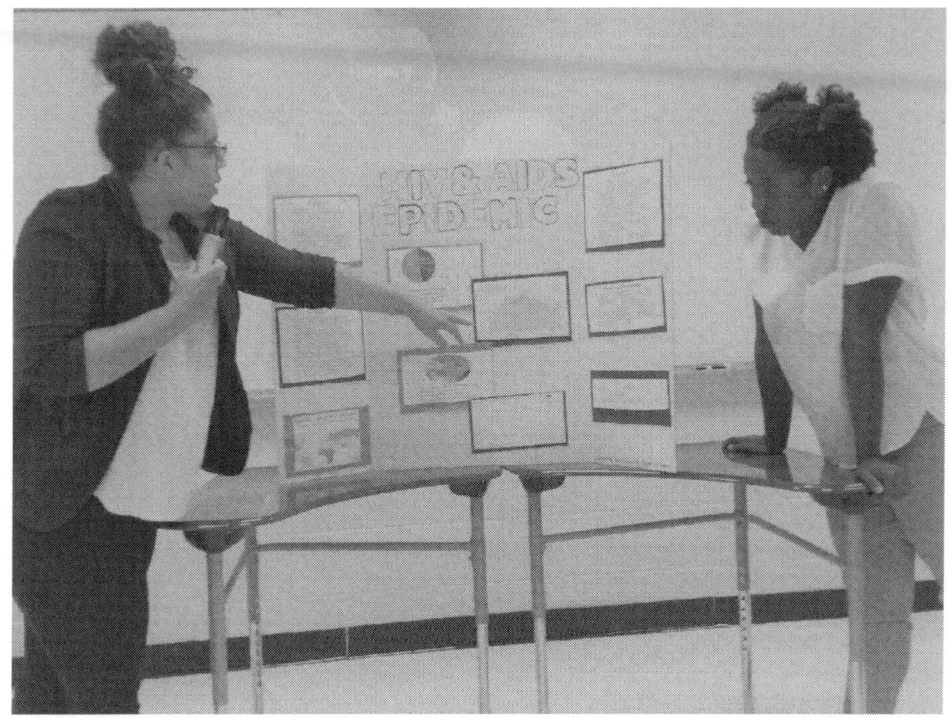


**Former Students Presents on HIV for Classroom Project**

HIPPA Laws provide privacy rights to patients. However, several insurance companies continued to deny preexisting conditions. Students can discuss real world issues while problem solving. Imagine an HIV patient trying to get health insurance during the early 1980s. Would they have been able to get coverage? What is ethical and what is the law?

Ethics directly describe the legal parameters of any project as well as the laws involved in testing a solution and or solving a community problem. Ethics may be considered as one of the most sensitive topics of epidemiology as it relates to religion, policies, culture, and social norms of a specific population. One must understand laws and policies before studying a specific outbreak as it determines and guides your practice for a solution. This unit teaches students how to apply principles of good ethical and legal practice as they research study designs, data collection, and dissemination of information as it relates to prevention of any outbreak. Ethical epidemiology teaches students the ethical and procedural methods as it relates to the law, how to collect and use public health data, and how to balance respect for individual privacy and risks of health threats to all community citizens. Students will understand how to apply public health codes as it relates to data collection, dissemination of information, and use of data. With that, students will learn the principles of justice, the role of timelines, and transparency of purpose when using public health information.

Unfortunately, some of the greatest milestones of scientific research were studies done unethically. The history of human science has always involved the use of animals for testing trials and experiment. Although it was illegal to use human subjects for test trials it was ethical to use African Americans as they were not viewed to be socially equal to European Americans. Even after slavery was abolished, several researchers within the science community continued to use black minorities for experimentation. As a result, several epidemics may have grown within the black community stemming from past unethical experimentation on African Americans.

Ethics of epidemiology is essential when describing the types of studies that can be used. What is ethical and what is unethical all depends on our society and how we view all cultures socially within our community.

In 1932 a study was done by the U.S. to diagnose the stages of syphilis on African American males in Tuskegee Alabama. The study was done on more than 400 African American men with syphilis to prove that we needed further research support and funds for a cure to syphilis. The men were given periodical exams and told they were being treated for bad blood. They were followed until their death as their health symptoms were only recorded instead of treated. In 1936 the decision to continue not treating and to follow the men until death was decided. https://www.cdc.gov/tuskegee/timeline.htm

This study was probably accepted by the public because in the early 1930's African Americans were not given basic civil rights as other Americans. Although using human subjects in test studies were against the law it was considered ethically accepted by researchers because it was again socially acceptable to view African Americans as second-class citizens to the majority. This does not excuse the behavior, yet it allows one to see how ethical standards affects a group of people.

Since this was a socially accepted norm it was considered ethical. Ethical standards were not in place until several years after the study was discontinued. Several programs and policies were implemented as a result of this long horrific past human experiment. I remember while sitting at the GHP during the summer of 1997 and hearing

President Clinton apologize live on television for the Tuskegee Syphilis experiment. I remember being shocked but not surprised. The Tuskegee University of National Center for Bioethics in Research and health care was formed along with several ethical standards and laws as a result of these unethical experiments.

Several other unethical studies were performed on African American Women. The HeLa Cells are historically known for its use in research in the development of understanding tissue regeneration. These cells were considered the first immortal cells obtained from an African American woman named Henrietta Lacks without her consent. Her cells were used for studies abroad for research without consent. The HeLa cells are still used today for cellular research. Her permission was not asked or considered in the quest for scientific advancements. https://www.hopkinsmedicine.org/henriettalacks/

There has been evidence for years of unethical treatment for African American women in science as some were treated as lab animals and not given anesthesia while being bound, gagged and cut for scientist to obtain tissue samples for research. Some scientist reported that negro women had a higher pain tolerance than white women as they witnessed firsthand how black women could withstand a higher tolerance for pain while performing surgery on them without medication. It is important for our students to understand the history both good and bad when learning science. Our students are intelligent enough to handle the truth.

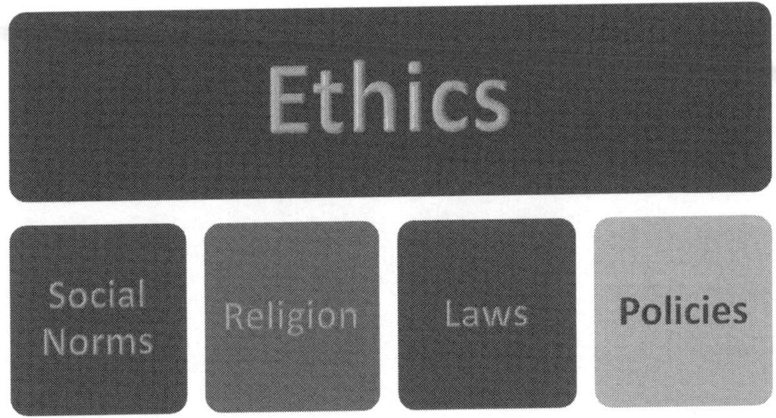


While researching ethics I come to understand the various categories of ethics. The one that caught my attention most was critical ethics. Critical Ethics is based on the needs within the community which may heavily depend on civil rights. The community must understand the priority of their specific needs as to others. For Example, in one community an epidemic may be an opioid epidemic while in another there could be a drag racing, homicide or suicide problem. The major public health concerns should be a part of the discussion as policies and laws are set for these communities.

**Framework 5 Public Health Surveillance and Solutions**:

Surveillance techniques allows students to evaluate their solutions to determine whether a specific solution works. This is where the students develop a solution and or scientific solution to the problem. In this unit, the students will understand how to disseminate findings from epidemiological research to the community or public health officials. Students will understand how public health agencies use surveillance data to describe and monitor health events in their jurisdictions. How this data is used to determine and identify any epidemic. How systemic practices may influence an epidemic. Students will learn the process for policy implementation and use these strategies in order to create programs, procedures, and laws that will promote good health. They will understand the importance of proper communication between health care providers, public health agencies, and the public. As well as the role of public health surveillance in policy and laws. Ethical standards are followed while students create innovative strategies and solutions. Students will also understand the role of various healthcare fields associated with public health policy and law.

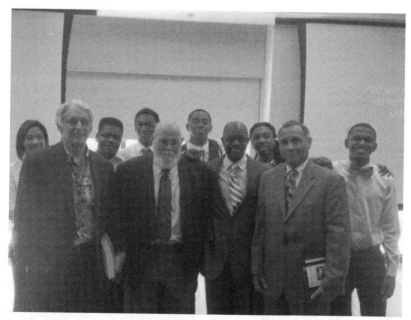

**David Kleinbaum, Ralph Cordell, Evern Williams, Juan Carlos and Students from Newton High School after Presenting at the Rollins School of Public Health Emory University**

Within the framework of public health surveillance, we will review analyze and discuss the value of current solutions to these problems. In 2012 the likelihood of death for all adults would be car accidents. A suggested solution to this problem by the Centers for Disease Control and Prevention was the implementation of the seatbelt safety law. Within the past ten years laws have been made to reduce the number of people dying in car accidents. This is an example of how public health influence the law. Also, over the past decade it has been made illegal to smoke cigarettes in a public restaurant and or bar. This law was largely pushed because of the research that proved secondhand smoke was just as harmful to the human body as firsthand smoke or worse.

Using the Five Frameworks

While teaching epidemiology and public health to students it is extremely important that they understand the importance and the characteristic of each of the five frameworks. They will need the framework for not just epidemiology but for basic problem solving and analyzing any problem. In an epidemiology class a student can solve a real-world problem with a real world researched based solution.

How to use the five frameworks teaching HIV to Epidemiology Students? Students will describe the five frameworks of epidemiology as it relates to HIV in America. Students must provide accurate information that will lead to a solution based on all the frameworks of epidemiology. They can later create or engineer possible solutions to these problems. Categorizing a large body of knowledge allows students to easily understand and make connections to various subjects within one specific problem. When teaching my students about the human immunodeficiency virus, I must provide them with a framework to categorize all the information received. The history of the HIV virus is important as it indicates the type of virus along with the time frame in which it became an epidemic within the United States. When teaching a lesson on HIV in America, we would first begin with the history of AIDS in America. The history of the HIV virus is important as it indicates the type of virus along with the time frame in which it became an epidemic within the United States. The instructor may want to discuss the history of retro viruses including the characteristics of the virus as well as how it affects the human body. Understanding the history of how the immune system responds to infections may be beneficial for the students to know the affects it has on the human body. When did this outbreak occur on American soil according to statistics and reports by the public health community?

Descriptive epidemiology identifies, person, place and time. What are the common characteristics of all the cases? In the early 1980's HIV was once called GRIDS, an acronym for gay related immune deficiency syndrome. This name was given based on the early diagnosis of individuals who first appeared to have the virus. The first cases shared some of the same characteristics. White homosexual males, between the age of 25 and 45 years of age living on opposite coast of the country, New York and San Francisco, CA. The name GRIDS was later changed to AIDS, acquired immune deficiency syndrome, because scientist later discovered that the virus could be contracted in several methods and to anyone. HIV is probably still the most popular virus known in the United States over the past 35 years.

When researching the ethics of HIV, students may learn of systemic barriers, along with ethical laws that derived from the outbreak of HIV. They may also learn of the ethical laws that affected the spread of the epidemic during that time. Blood banks did not screen for HIV during the epidemic in the early 1980's. Also, one may remember how football players could wear a bloody jersey and stay in the game. The onset of a deadly virus able to transfer from one human to another with blood contact was enough to cause a shockwave of changes throughout the country as it related to health precautions in handling blood.

Public health surveillance of solutions, surveys data and solutions to determine what is currently used as a solution and what affect does it have on solving the problem. After getting this information they must then decide how to disseminate this information to the public. The use of information from all previous frameworks are used as a resource for testing and comparing data. Public health surveillance also makes recommendations for policies aimed at reducing an epidemic. Surveillance identified that more effective screening of HIV by blood banks and the increase of education as a preventative method. As public health crisis continues to be a problem within the world every attempt and opportunity to save a life and reduce the spread of an infections is a step towards a healthier world.

Since all epidemics are data driven, it allows teachers to deliver the topic from an analytical point of view instead of a personal viewpoint. Everyone living has experienced losing a loved one from either a tragic event, chronic illness, or infectious disease. When the topic of epidemiology covers such a broad range of topics it gives interest to a larger population of students which crosses racial, social, religious and cultural differences. They gain an understanding of how certain epidemics are more prevalent within certain subgroups. These subgroups are represented by various cultures. This leads to conversations and discussions that will enhance a student and teachers' cultural awareness. The epidemic of prostate cancer, opioid addiction and Zika virus are great lesson topics that will allow for such cultural awareness and educational opportunities.

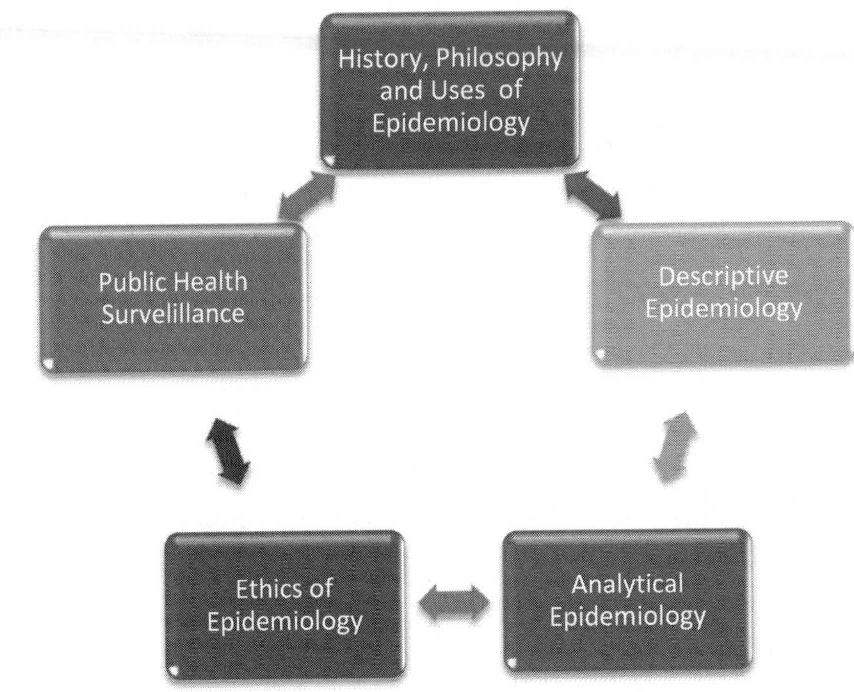
History, Philosophy and Uses of Epidemiology
Public Health Survelillance
Descriptive Epidemiology
Ethics of Epidemiology
Analytical Epidemiology

# 10

# Research Is Real

There is no one program that defines the way in which epidemiology and public health fits directly under the umbrella of public education. It is the approach to the subject of epidemiology that shows a true connection to local, state, and federal guidelines that are necessary for academic success. Epidemiology has all the three R's of education. Rigor, Relevance, and it helps build Relationships. Teachers may easily work together as they take their students through various aspects of the problem-solving framework

One of the most intriguing aspects of teaching for me was the opportunity to always learn new strategies and teaching methodologies. Blooms taxonomy, Marzano's Strategies and Daggett's four quadrants are a few strategies that several school districts have adopted. In the efforts of making my classroom curriculum, I would always try to make my topics relevant to something in the real world. I found that this was one of the few ways to keep my students interested in the curriculum. The strategies allowed me to demonstrate and organize my lessons to colleagues and supervisors. Teachers need to be competent with both their content and their abilities within the classroom in order to tie subject matter to research based instructional strategies. They must also be able to reach all students and continuously accept new ideas and strategies as time brings on a different type of student and or issue.

Blooms Taxonomy, developed by Benjamin Bloom along with collaborators Max Englehawort and Edward Furst, David Krathwohl and Walter Hill published a framework for identifying educational goals. The framework includes a pyramid of words that describe the essential needs for student success. https://www.bloomstaxonomy.net/

Create, evaluate, analyze, apply, understand, and remember. Students love to have the opportunity to discuss, create and evaluate real world problems. They are more observant and critical of our environment than we think. Topics and curriculums focused on public health problems provide students the opportunity to use critical thinking skills for everyday problems. Blooms taxonomy, and Marzano's strategy is easily demonstrated within the curriculum of epidemiology. Marzano's nine strategies for effective teaching is another one of the most used strategies by educators within my district and surrounding counties. Teachers have no problem understanding the strategies however, when covering all the topics within the curriculum, some teachers struggle to utilize all the strategies. On the other hand, many teachers have the "I DO THAT MOMENT, while attending a conference. You may practice something by habit without knowing it is a research based instructional strategy. Teaching epidemiology enables educators the opportunity to effectively use the following Marzano's strategies

Robertos Marzano's Nine effective Instructional Strategies,

1. Identifying similarities and differences
2. Summarizing and note taking
3. Reinforcing Effort and Providing Feedback
4. Homework and Practice
5. Nonlinguistic Representation
6. Cooperative Learning
7. Setting Objectives and Providing Feedback
8. Generating and Testing Hypothesis
9. Cues, Questions, and Advance Organizers

https://www.teachthought.com/learning/marzanos-9-instructional-strategies-graphic/

.

While learning the competencies of epidemiology and public health a student must continue to make comparisons and identify similarities and differences. Some case studies will allow students to compare similarities and differences between groups within populations. This is a common practice of epidemiologist and researchers.

Summarizing, note taking, setting objectives and providing feedback is annotated by the description of a specific outbreak. To describe person place and time one must practice detailed summary reports with specific information regarding cases. The public health surveillance strategies will educate students on how to disseminate this information in a proper and legal way.

Reinforcing effort and providing feedback is a common practice during public health surveillance and testing solutions. There may be variables that may affect a specific number. For example, if students must decrease the spread of infection in a school, they would make necessary changes and or provide solutions to these problems. They must evaluate their solution by determining if the solution was successful in reducing the numbers by using the proper research methods. Students can perform experiments within the field of public health and epidemiology. Experiments on reducing the spread of the flu in the school can give them a hands-on approach to problem solving. Microbiology and disease detective labs provide students the opportunity to simulate careers in public health.

Before doing the experiment, they must get all the information and data of infected students and or absences due to illness during the flu season. The comparison of the attendance may be a logical data base comparing absences from one year to the next during the flu season. Students may develop habits of cleaning surfaces, washing hands more regularly and reduce personal contact with those showing signs of infection.

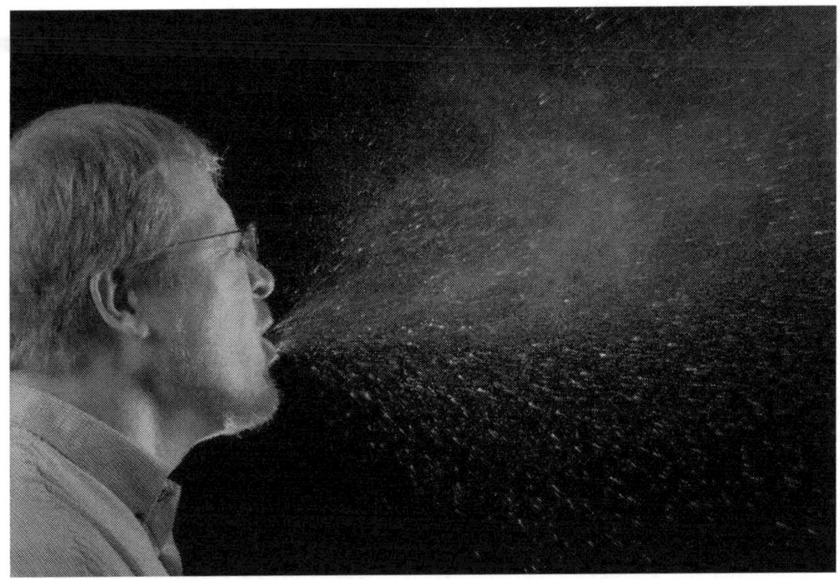

https://en.wikipedia.org/wiki/File:Sneeze.JPG

Non-Linguistic; would be demonstrated by the tri board projects describing the Five Frameworks of Epidemiology.

The students may work in groups, pairs or individually. Students choosing to work in a group may decide to present on a specific topic from the framework while allowing their partners to present the other topics. Collaborative learning allows students to begin building positive educational and business relationships with one another.

Students generate and test hypothesis constantly brainstorming to figure out solutions to the problem. When the primary purpose of both epidemiologist and doctors are to save lives, students should first know what is causing the problem. Not only do we need to understand what is destroying us, but we also need to know the most known preventive strategies that may decrease chances of becoming ill. All solutions eventually will need to be tested when following the scientific method. The scientific method is described as the steps methods and procedures utilized to solve a scientific problem. Within every scientific method there is an experiment. An experiment bound by ethics and standards that must be followed. By working on scientific experiments and projects students are afforded the opportunity to experience how ethical guidelines and policies may shape the limits of their projects.

Daggett's strategies emphasize knowledge taxonomy, evaluate, synthesis, analysis, application comprehension and knowledge awareness. Students constantly can make connections to real world problems by studying public health issues. The quadrants are assimilation, acquisition, adaptation and application. These quadrants describe a process of teaching students how to obtain, learn and adapt to the environment with the information received from a specific lesson.

www.daggett.com/pdf/Quadrant_D_Leadership_2014.pdf

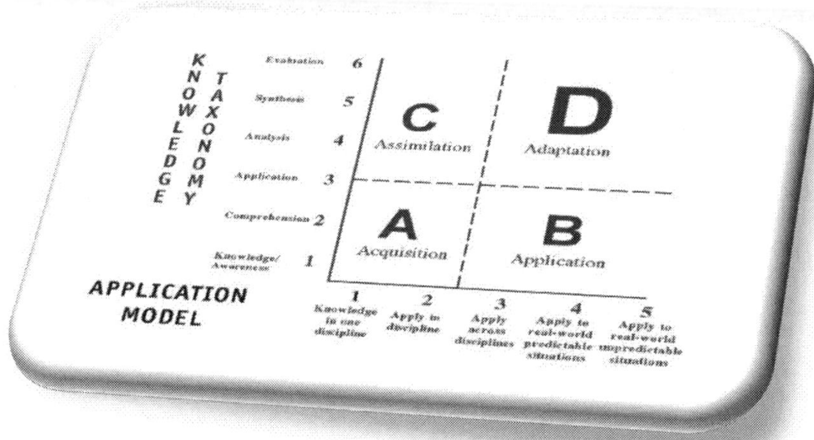


The objective here is to teach teachers how to make connections with the real world and inspire students to learn enough information that he or she will modify their behaviors and actions based on the information learned during a lesson. What if the topic of discussion within the classroom limits the ability of the student to be creative? As we know, everyone is different and has different interest. The four quadrants provide teachers with a guide for connecting the subject with the student. Quadrant A is Acquisition, acquiring the information from the instructor. Quadrant B is Application, how do you apply the knowledge from the instructor. Quadrant C is Assimilation, and D is Adaptation. Assimilation is the process in which a student's takes all this information in and really understand it. While Adaptation is defined as the evolutionary process in which an organism becomes better able to live in its environment. Epidemiology provides topics that will encourage students how to modify their behaviors in order to maintain a safer and healthier lifestyle. The five frameworks can provide the students with a model that will give them the ability to easily identify and successfully cover all the four quadrants. It may also assist in making connections and allows for a more realistic connection with life and other subjects. How have we adapted to the long-term effects of the coronavirus outbreak. Will most of us ever think the same again about germs and viruses? Will there be precautionary measures taken differently after the pandemic?

Beyond the research based instructional strategies you must follow the guidelines of educational scholars, as well as state, and national standards. The very thought of this sounded intimidating at first however, the five frameworks aligned and fit like a key with Mark Kaelins Enduring Epidemiological Understandings, Georgia Science Standards and the National Science Standards.

The enduring understandings of Epidemiology was developed by Dr. Mark Kaelin and Dr. Wendy Huebner, and Dr. Ralph Cordell. Along with educators across the country these enduring understandings each fall under one of the five framework umbrellas.

**ENDURING UNDERSTANDINGS**

These are the big ideas of a discipline that have lasting value outside the classroom. The table below shows another version of epidemiology component and the enduring understandings for each one.

**Overarching Epidemiological Concept**

**History:** 1. The causes of health and disease are discoverable by systematically and rigorously identifying their patterns in populations, formulating causal hypotheses, and testing those hypotheses by making group comparisons. These methods lie at the core of the science of epidemiology. Epidemiology is the basic science of public health, a discipline responsible for improving health and preventing disease in populations.

## Identifying Patterns of Health and Disease and Formulating Hypotheses

**Public Health Surveillance**: 2. Health and disease are not distributed haphazardly in a population. There are patterns to their occurrence. These patterns can be identified through the surveillance of populations.

**Analytical, Descriptive:** 3. **Analysis of these patterns can help formulate hypotheses about the possible causes of health and** disease.

## Making Group Comparisons and Identifying Associations

**Analytical: 4** A hypothesis can be tested by comparing the frequency of disease in selected groups of people with and without an exposure to determine if the exposure and the disease are associated.

**Ethics: 5** When an exposure is hypothesized to have a beneficial effect, studies can be designed in which a group of people is intentionally exposed to the hypothesized cause and compared to a group that is not exposed.

**Ethics:** 6 When an exposure is hypothesized to have a detrimental effect, it is not ethical to intentionally expose a group of people. In these circumstances, studies can be designed that observe groups of free-living people with and without the exposure.

## Explaining Associations and Judging Causation

**Descriptive**: 7. One possible explanation for finding an association is that the exposure causes the outcome. Because studies are complicated by factors not controlled by the observer, other explanations also must be considered, including confounding, chance and bias.

**Ethics, Descriptive:** 8. While a given exposure may be necessary to cause an outcome, the presence of a single factor is seldom enough. Most outcomes are caused by a combination of exposures that may include genetic make-up, behaviors, social, economic, and cultural factors and the environment.

**Public Health Surveillance:** **9** Judgments about whether an exposure causes a disease are developed by examining a body of epidemiologic evidence as well as evidence from other scientific disciplines.

## Improving Health and Preventing Disease

**Ethics**: 10. Individual and societal health-related decisions to improve health and prevent disease are based on more than scientific evidence. Social, economic, ethical, environmental, cultural, and political factors may also be considered in decision-making.

**Public Health Surveillance:** 11. effectiveness of a health-related strategy can be evaluated by comparing the frequency of disease in selected groups of people who were and were not exposed to the strategy. Costs, trade-offs, and alternative solutions must also be considered in evaluating the strategy.

## Understanding Non-Health Related Phenomena

**History and Philosophy:** **12** An understanding of non-health related phenomena can be developed through epidemiologic thinking, by identifying their patterns in populations, formulating causal hypotheses, and testing those hypotheses by making group comparisons.

http://www.epiedmovement.org/BMEU.html

Georgia Science Standards:

The state of Georgia standards for science teachers based on the Georgia Standards for Excellence. These standards are Clarification, Practices and Cross Cutting concepts, Increased Rigor and Foundation for STEM and Literacy Integration. Providing a curriculum of public health and epidemiology gives students a clear identification of all of the various standards for both the each of these areas. Practice, is a description of behaviors and strategies that scientist use while they investigate and create solutions to problems. This is a common practice among public health investigators as they continue to solve problems that may affect our population. Cross cutting is another standard that is common amongst the scientific community as it allows for students to relate a specific topic to a much broader field of sciences.

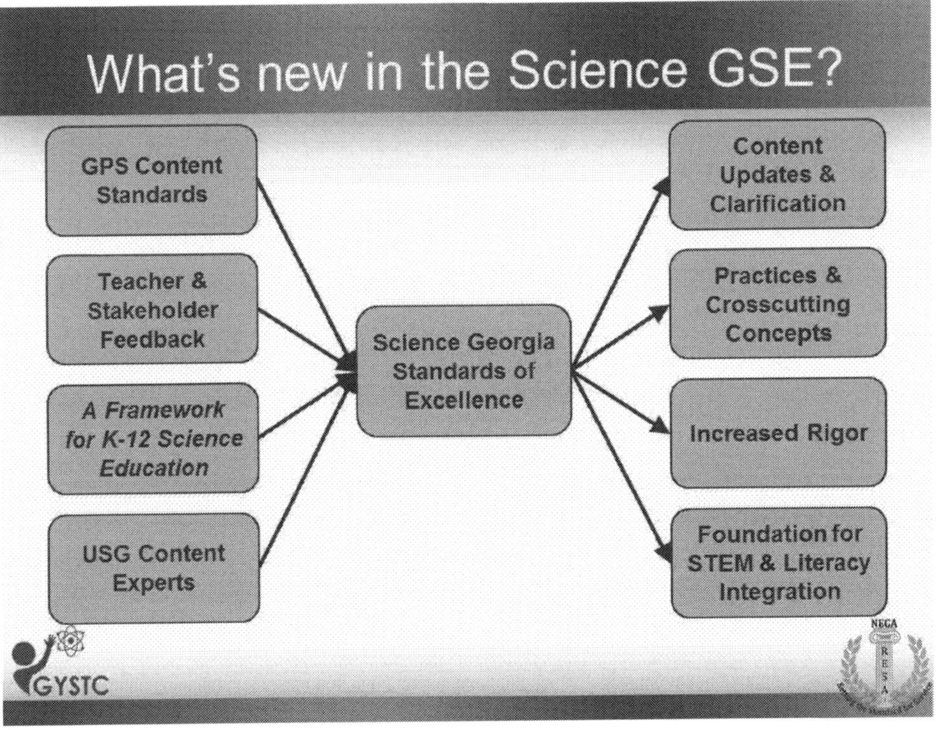


http://www.negaresa.org/science/wp-content/uploads/2016/07/Slide5.jpg

Some investigations may involve a variety of subjects ranging from , zoology, to math to social sciences. Engaging students as investigators provides them the opportunity to see how all subjects may be used in solving a real world health crisis. The swine flu, a respiratory influenza virus found in pigs that somehow made its way into the human population over ten years ago. As any other virus there are different strains as the one which affected the human population in 2009 was described as the H1N1 virus. Since the virus originates in pigs, we can easily see how epidemiologist utilize other professions and topics such as zoology and veterinarian science.

The Next Generation Science Standards are the guides for what the students should know and do for science k-12 subjects nationally. These standards are divided into three primary areas, Practice, Core Ideas and Crosscutting. Practice involves the actual actions and protocol scientist follow to investigate problems and build sollutions. Crosscutting shows how concepts require scientist and problem solvers to include multiple disciplines including several subjects both science and non science.

**Next Generation Science Standards; Practices, Core Ideas, and Cross Cutting**

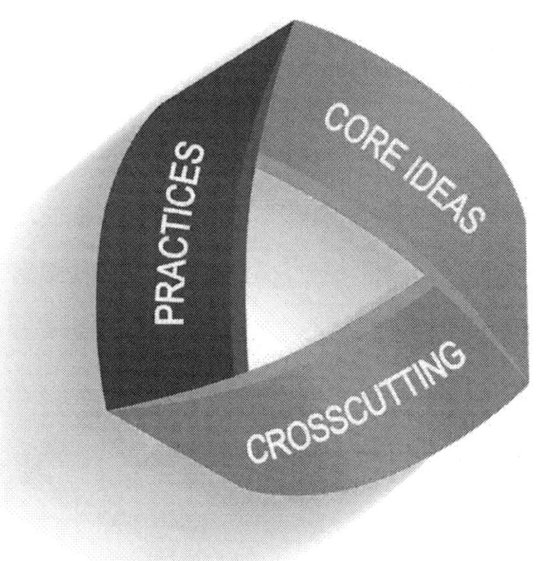


https://www.nextgenscience.org/

The disciplinary core ideas are broken into three primary areas for all science grade levels k-12, Life Science, Earth and Space Science and Physical Science. Epidemiology is definitely a subject that involves all three of the core ideas as well as cross cutting and practice. While creating new inventions and solutions to problems, such as engineering. Physical science is covered in a more practical hands on approach to create new solutions. This strategy is used when guiding students to create and engineer models of proposed physical solutions to everyday problems.

Content or the discipline core idea, have broad importance across multiple sciences or displines as part of a single subject. This provides students another example of how public health covers a wider range of professions including engineering.

Public Health studies increases rigor in STEM and Literacy. Students have the opportuniy to read, research and create solutions to specific problems

Rigor, relevance and relationships are commonly heard terms that serves as a guiding framework to student achievement. Rigor is defined as a measure of depth in understanding. *{www.edutopia.org/blog/a-new-definition-of-rigor}.* Relevance is defined as the state of being intricately connected or appropriate for a current situation. Are the topics we teach in school relevant to real world problems we may deal with in our society? All topics selected and discussed in public health has an outcome that may result in deaths of individuals. Several of the case studies, topics and statistics studied are from real outbreak investigations. Relationships are important in developing and creating a healthy learning environment. One of the most important characteristics of a successful educator is to have excellent listening skills. Although several may not want to put emphasis on this topic it is essential if we really want to hear our students and community. Providing opportunities for students and instructors to have open discussions on community epidemics allows both the instructor and student the opportunity to build a positive relationship based on similar experiences.

Epidemiology and Public Health is Rigorous

Epidemiology allows students to utilize critical thinking skills along with analyzing data and interpreting model solutions. Rigor is described by educators as a teaching practice that requires the students to think critically and apply the knowledge that they learn rather than just memorizing the material. The students will be able to think much deeper and provide possible solutions to solve specific social and health problems.

Advanced classes are commonly considered rigorous because of the amount of work given to the student and the amount of information the student is required to recall. On the other hand, rigor may be considered the ability of the student to see the relevance and use critical thinking skills to solve problems.

Relevance

Every student has lost a loved one to at least one epidemic. With such a broad range of topics and subjects in epidemiology and public health there is a strong possibility that one or more epidemics has hit close to home. Students seem to be more relaxed, motivated and comfortable discussing topics that they may have some experience with. The thought of thinking in a way that may solve an everyday problem may excite some students. Community leaders may want to visit classrooms during some discussions. The problems are real, and the data is accurate. Real community problems and possible solutions presented by students. Providing students, the opportunity to present these community problems theories and solutions created from research is a wonderful opportunity for students to connect with community members and scholars.

Relationships

Students can become exposed to several different career fields. They also meet scholars from the professional and educational fields epidemiology and public health.

**PRESS RELEASE/Invitation**

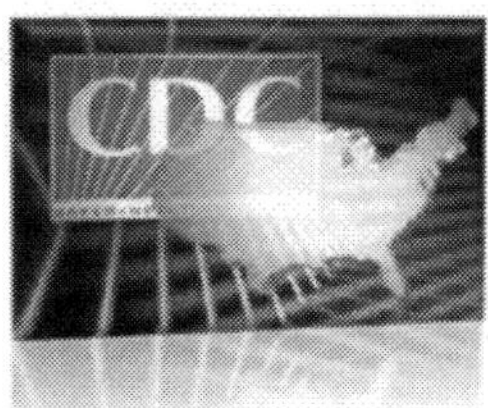


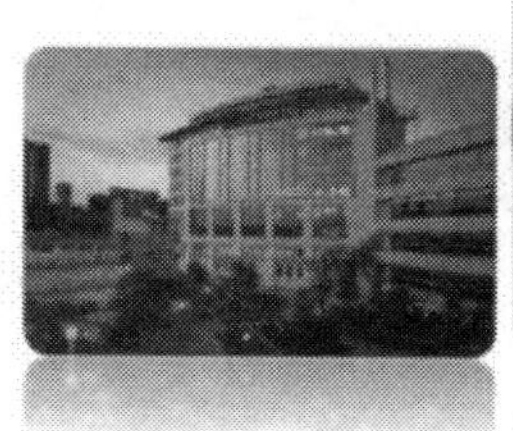

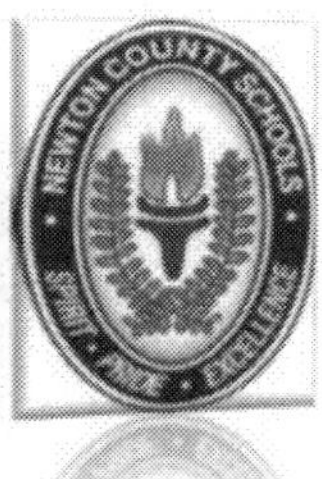


**FOR IMMEDIATE RELEASE**
**SEPTEMBER 25, 2013**

## Teaching Epidemiology in Public Schools

**STEM Innovation of Math and Science/Real World Application of Biostatistics**

**When:** September 27th 2013

**Where:** The Rollins School of Public Health
Lawrence P. and Ann Estes Klamon room
Claudia Nance Rollins Building, Room 8030
1518 Clifton Rd. NE
Atlanta GA 30309

**Time:** 10:00 am to 12:00noon

**Public Health and Educational Speakers include:**

**Mr. Evern Williams, *Pioneer, Epidemiology Educationalist***
**Newton High School**

**Dr. James W. Curran, *Dean***
**Rollins School of Public Health**

**Dr. Ralph Cordell**
**OSELS/SEPDPO/CDC**

**Dr. David Kleinbaum, *Professor***
**Emory University**

**Mr. John Ellenberg, *Assistant Principal***
**Newton High School**

**Dr. Juan Carlos-Aguilar, *Science Program Manager***
**Division of Curriculum and Instruction, Georgia Department of Education**

.

The CDC currently has the High School Public Health and Epidemiology Core Competency

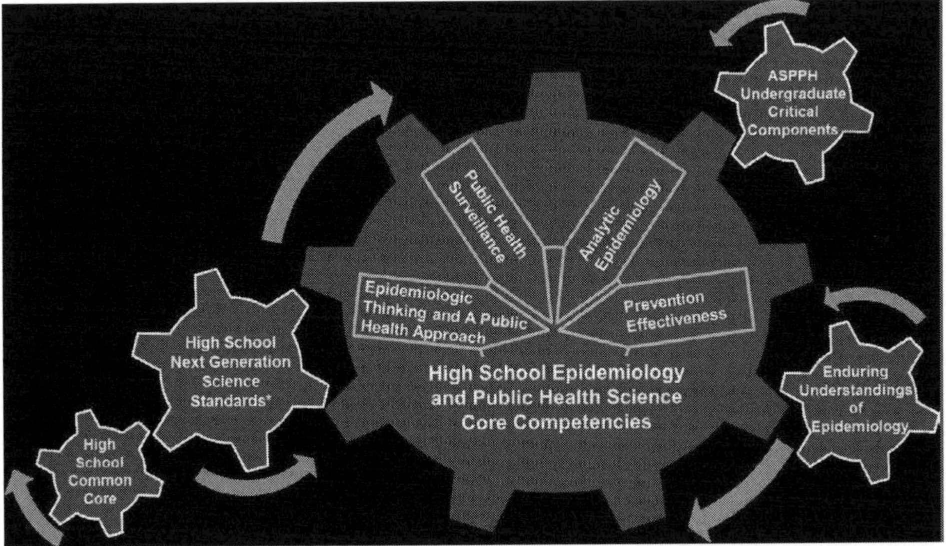


https://www.cdc.gov/careerpaths/k12teacherroadmap/pdfs/ephs-competencies.pdf

The CDC currently offers High School Epidemiology and Public Health Science Core Competencies. I was also instrumental in developing this tool as it started out as the Five Frameworks for teaching high school epidemiology.

Dr. Ralph Cordell and I began the work under the leadership of the late Dr. Stephen B. Thacker. These competencies assist in teaching the topic of epidemiology as an extra unit in some science classes.

The five frameworks designed for teaching epidemiology eventually evolved into the core competencies of epidemiology and public health. I designed the five frameworks to enable students to engage in a year-long class. I continued to train educators, students and community leaders throughout the state on how to teach public health based on the framework. Most had the same response, "It was easy to follow and understand and puts things in perspective". Epidemiology provides little boundaries as it pertains to the various components of education and subjects that all pertain to real life.

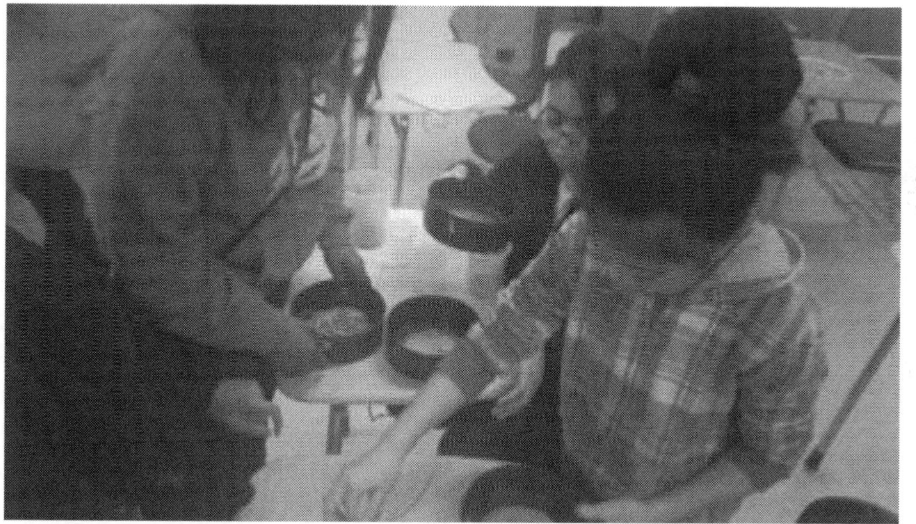

Middle School Students working on Epidemiology Project.

# 11

# United by Epi

Currently curriculum integration is one of the most sought-after strategies for teaching. What exactly is curriculum integration? In its most simple description, it is about making connections to students' real lives with knowledge that can be embedded into multiple disciplines. Many state and national educational standards recognize curriculum integration or cross cutting as an important part of education.

STEM (Science, Technology, Engineering, and Math) programs provide meaningful platforms for students to express what they have learned in multiple ways. It has continued to gain popularity and has been utilized as part of differentiated services for the past ten years. Epidemiology could easily be integrated into existing STEM programs. Exemplary STEM teachers engage and collaborate within and across disciplines when organizing content units. Teachers are encouraged to engage higher order thinking skills by creating more explicit opportunities for students to apply new skill sets. One example is project-based learning.

While the objective of STEM is to develop students' ability to solve problems; seek evidence or supporting information, and know how to evaluate evidence for validity; The long lasting goal of teaching

Epidemiology in schools is to help students and their families make healthier decisions. It is easy, feels good teaching, and fits well into existing teaching models especially for those looking for a boost in student energy by using curriculum integration strategies in their classrooms. Here is a diagram I created which demonstrates how epidemiology framework was used in all subjects in a high school and middle school. Portions of the framework were adapted and then tested in elementary school environments.

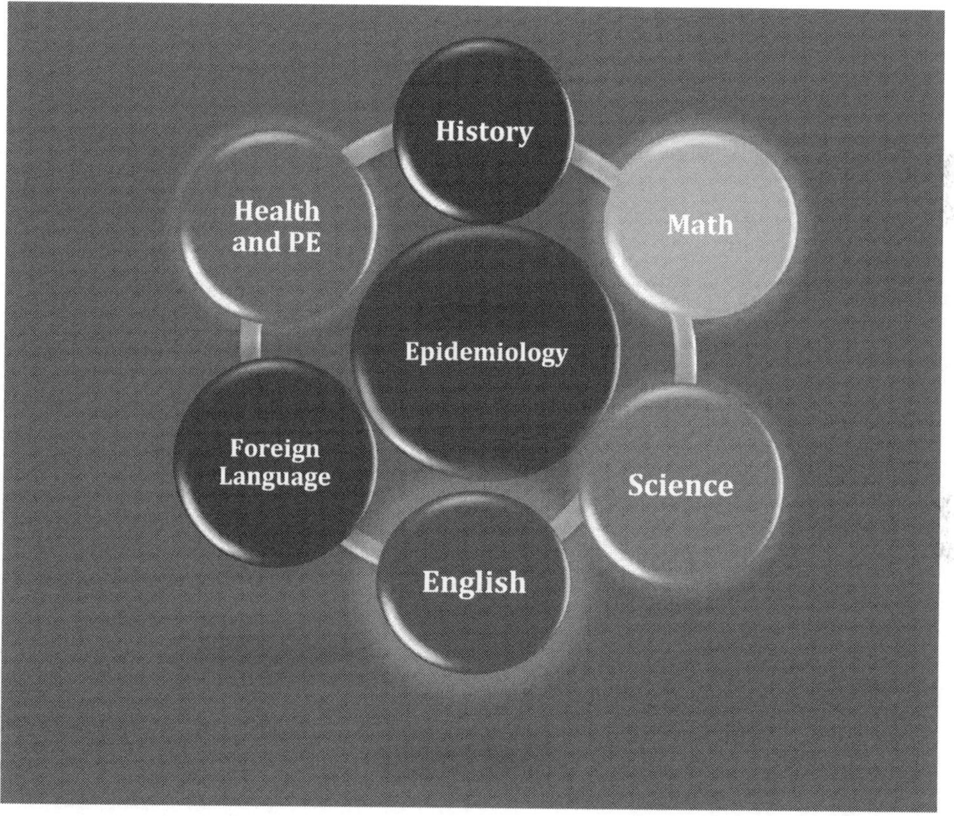


Epidemiology builds a bridge around all subjects. Students apply concepts from other classes through collaborative professional learning activities. Teachers work as a team by planning and sharing student feedback; These healthy teaching practices engage both teachers and students' opportunities to learn together and identify specific problems and creating solutions as part of a community. Community visions need full circle supports and differentiated services that matter.

. Epi is a gateway for you to practice teaching strategies while helping families in need, why not have students solve the problems of tomorrow, Future student investments begin with heightened interest in solving real world problems to find solutions. I constantly remind my students that it only takes one invention, policy change, or cure to save thousands of lives.

The historical perspective of any disease is built into the framework. Allow students to display created information with references after studying the case history of a disease related problem. A slice of this pie could be taught in various classes. Science, Math, History, or Language Arts as students show how diseases affect individuals and populations by assimilation. The history of past outbreaks such as the bubonic plaque, smallpox and the flu are all infectious diseases and epidemics which have shaped history. Science investigators participate in labs that simulate a real-world outbreak and report on findings. Biology might expand on describing the lifecycle and identifying structures of the various types of viruses. The successful integration of curriculum with key aspects of teaching with various subjects in the study of diseases is possible. The CDC decided to name the teaching module EXCITE, an acronym for Excellence in Curriculum Integration through Teaching Epidemiology. EXCITE served as a teaching model for middle and high school teachers from

1997 to 2017. It is currently named the career paths to public health. Add link to the site?

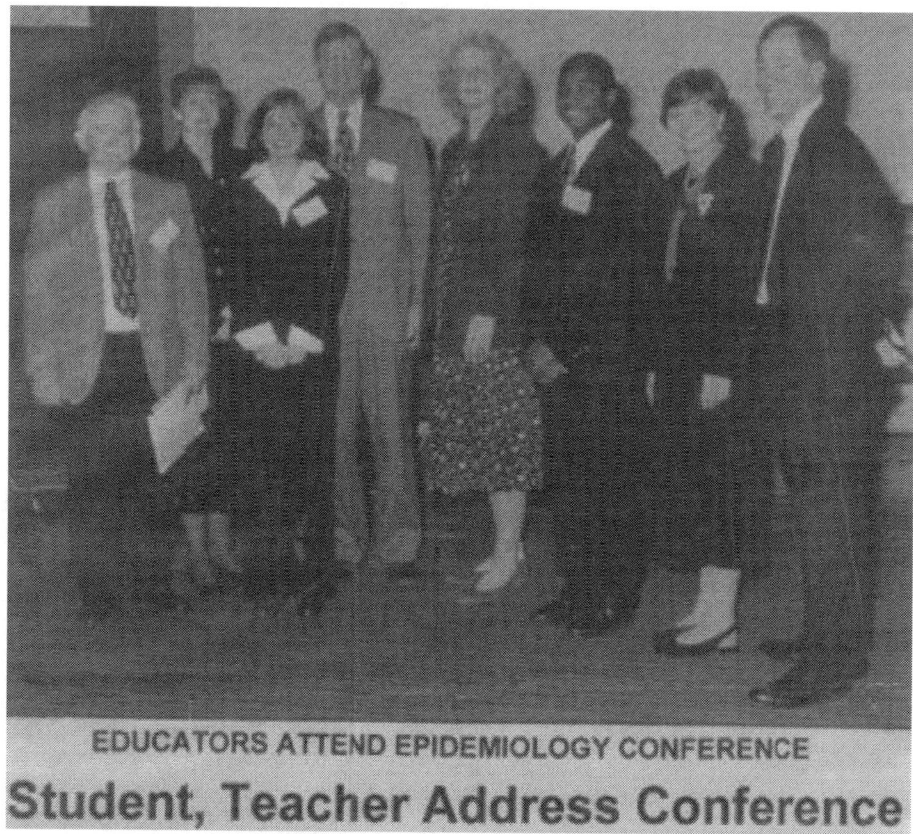
EDUCATORS ATTEND EPIDEMIOLOGY CONFERENCE

**Student, Teacher Address Conference**

Dr. Julian Cope, Mrs. Sara Hayes, Ms. Tara Hayes, Mr. Jimmy Jordan, Dr. Claire Broone, Mr. Evern Williams, Dr. Donna Stroup, Dr. Stephen B. Thacker.

Epidemiology Program Conference Presentation 1998

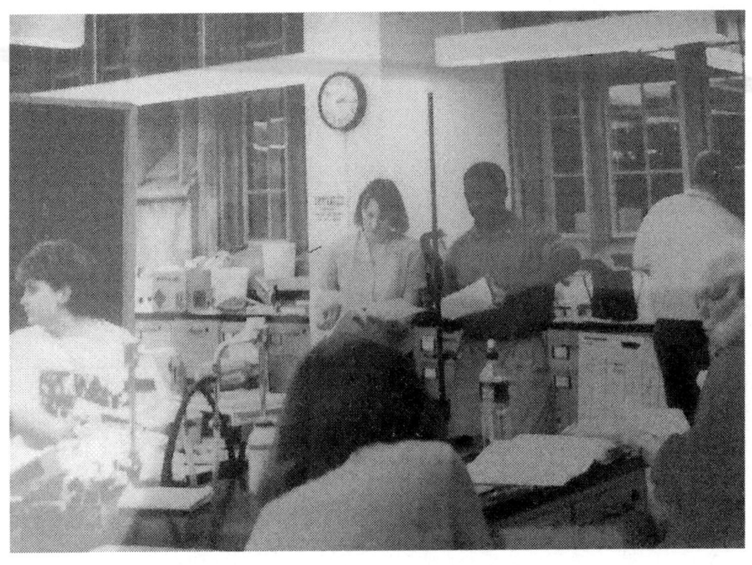

Dr. Ruth Berkelmen and Evern Williams, Teaching at Princeton University, Woodrow Wilson Institute for Teachers, 1997

After September 11, 2001, there seemed to be less attention to teaching epidemiology to students and more on bioterrorism. Several other professors went on to obtain grants from various organizations aimed at providing students with epidemiology curriculum. In 2000 I was promoted from the classroom to the Director of Alternative Schools for the Jasper county school system. My students were the first in the county who had to wear uniforms in high school. I was strict with them as they were in alternative school for a reason. The environment was structured but fair. In the design of the curriculum we used the principals of epidemiology methods with our students that provided real world scenarios. Our staff provided an environment that allowed students to speak openly and honestly about real world problems. At the time, EXCITE, served as the educational module for educators for the CDC. The students knew that I was directly involved in the development of that program. Several links on the internet revealed speaking engagements from universities such as Princeton University, Emory University, and University of Georgia. Years later several of these URL's would be deleted or removed by the owners.

The students had immediate respect for me as they knew and saw someone working with them that they felt could work anywhere. As a result, the students began to understand procedures, policies, laws and how their reactions to scenarios affect their overall outcome. They joined the FFA and were one of the first schools in the state of Georgia to participate in composting their lunch waste. The program was headed by the University of Georgia and the FFA organization in Monticello. A graduate student from University of Georgia worked with our school on the project and suggested that the students visit the University of Georgia's, agriculture department and view how composting was done on a larger scale. I remember when I put in a recommendation for my alternative students to visit UGA my supervisor was shocked. I guess most people would think twice about taking a group of students from an alternative school to the University of Georgia. For fear that some may become disruptive or cause problems. I knew that each of these students needed an outlet. They learned soft skills and respect for their community and were always seen doing something to help the city. They began to volunteer in the community with the chamber of commerce and were commonly seen in the community by their peers and former teachers. The trip was a success without a single problem with an article in the local newspaper describing the trip. Several of those students have gone on to live successful and productive lives.

From 2004-2006 more of the work I did as a consultant was replaced by college professors and grants to enhance the platform of EXCITE. There was no known potential pandemic at that time. From 2006 to 2009 I worked in Newton County Schools as a science teacher and 7th grade team leader in one of the middle schools. In 2009 H1N1 became a health threat and potential epidemic or pandemic.

I contacted Dr. Stephen B. Thacker from the CDC whom I had previously consulted for in earlier years. I remember asking Dr. Thacker if he remembered me and he stated, "of course I remember you Evern". I discussed the idea of me designing a curriculum for the CDC that will enable students to learn how to prevent the spread of H1N1 flu in schools without interfering with the normal learning curriculum and standards necessary for each class. Dr. Thacker agreed to allow me to design the curriculum to help prevent the spread of the flu.

The curriculum was designed to decrease the spread of the flu in schools. Students learn both the morphology of the virus and how it is spread. As well as the most preventive strategies used to reduce the spread of a virus.

I have always told my students that a virus is not considered a living organism because it does not have all the characteristics of what scientist define as life. Although it may possess the characteristics of life it will probably be the most threatening force against the human species.

One may ask how to do you began to design a lesson plan for all these subjects. The objective was to get as many subjects involved in this one topic as possible. And to get them to teach the topic on the same day or days within the same week. After about three months the curriculum was complete as representatives from the CDC, Georgia State Department of Education and Georgia Bio took a day to come visit the teachers at Newton High School present the unit. The title of the integrating unit was FLU EXIT, an acronym for Educational eXcellence through Integrative Teaching. The visit resulted in great reviews, some calling it one of the best representations of curriculum integration that they had ever seen.

I have provided an example of the lesson with Biology, Spanish and History class. The school project provides lesson plans for more than 13 different subjects. I replaced the H1N1 virus with the Coronavirus within the book to provide a much more relevant topic.

# *FLU EXIT*

***Educational eXcellence through Integrative Teaching***

## *History*

Essential Question: How much of an impact has viruses had on the development of America?
Ask students what do they know about the Coronavirus?
Allow students to discuss the various things they may have heard in the media before showing the power point

Flu Activity:
Coronavirus Activity

While the Covid-19 ravages much of China and world leaders rush to close their borders to protect citizens from the outbreak, the flu has quietly killed 10,000 in the U.S. so far this influenza season.

At least 19 million people have come down with the flu in the U.S. with 180,000 ending up in the hospital, according to the Centers for Disease Control and Prevention. The flu season, which started in September and can run until May, is currently at its peak and poses a greater health threat to the U.S. than the new coronavirus, physicians say. The new virus, which first emerged in Wuhan, China, on Dec. 31, has sickened roughly 17,400 and killed 362 people mostly in that country as of Monday morning.

Allow student to read article on the recent Coronavirus,

Discuss the article with students; How did the resent outbreak begin?

Discuss the Flu Epidemic of 1918 which killed more than 21 Million people.

See how viruses and plagues of the present and past has shaped our culture.

Make sure students understand how to prevent the spread of the FLU along with the symptoms.

1.) **Brief History**
2.) **Symptoms**
3.) **Treatment**
4.) **How to Prevent the Spread of Influenza**

Students will make a current Spot Map by indicating state, national or international outbreaks.

# Biology

## Background

CDC is responding to an outbreak of respiratory disease caused by a novel (new) coronavirus that was first detected in China and which has now been detected in more than 100 locations internationally, including in the United States. The virus has been named "SARS-CoV-2" and the disease it causes has been named "coronavirus disease 2019" (abbreviated "COVID-19").

On January 30, 2020, the International Health Regulations Emergency Committee of the World Health Organization (WHO) declared the outbreak ``" (PHEIC). On January 31, Health and Human Services Secretary Alex M. Azar II declared a public health emergency (PHE) for the United States to aid the nation's healthcare community in responding to COVID-19. On March 11, WHO publicly external icon characterized COVID-19 as a pandemic. On March 13, the President of the United States declared the COVID-19 outbreak a national emergency.

**Flu Activity:** According to the May 9-May 15, 2010 Flu View, flu activity in the United States declined again from the previous week. Flu activity is low nationwide with only a small number of influenza viruses being reported, most of which were 2009 H1N1. Flu is unpredictable, but sporadic cases of flu, caused by either 2009 H1N1 or seasonal flu viruses, will likely continue to occur throughout the spring and summer in the United States. Internationally, 2009 H1N1 viruses are still circulating, including in the Southern Hemisphere, which is entering its flu season. For more information, please see the international situation update

While all the classes received information on specific aspects of the virus, all received knowledge on how to prevent the spread of an outbreak.

- Wash your hands as often as you can.
- If your sick stay at home
- Policies in place to keep those showing flu symptoms home
- Keep your distance away from those in public
- Wipe door knobs off and items commonly touched by the public clean
- Eat healthy drink plenty of vitamin C.
- Cover your mouth when you cough, or wear a mask to prevent infection
- Prevent from touching others especially handshakes
- Get Vaccinated
- Stay alert and current with accurate information from a reliable source

**Essential Question.**
**What is COVID-19 or Influenza virus and how can we prevent it from spreading?**

**Ask students what do they know about any flu virus?**
Allow students to discuss the various things they may have heard in the media before showing the power point.

Please use the Slides for the Lecture. There are approximately 12 - 14 slides that will emphasize the principles of epidemiology along with teaching students the basic characteristics of the Virus.
After the power point allow students to search the CDC website to view the various types of Viruses. www.cdc.gov after going to the site the students should type in the word Virus Diagrams
The students will get into groups of three to four and began constructing a three-dimensional model of the H1N1 or COVID-19.
The model should include.
**Hemagglutinin**, - Bonding Protein
**Glycoprotein spike**- enzyme that breaks down the cell wall.
**Capsid-**
**RNA-**

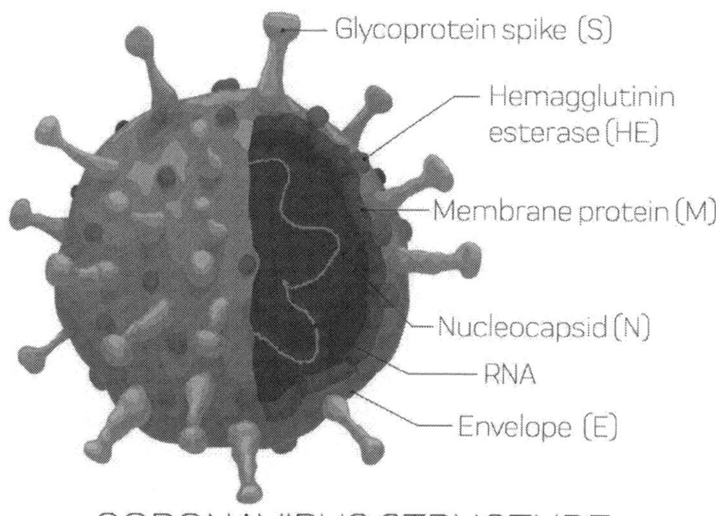


https://www.google.com/search?q=coronavirus+labeled+diagram&source=lnms&tbm

All students will have the same material and construct the models with the material available.
The models should be completed before class ends.
Students you will create a three-dimensional Model of the COVID-19 Virus.
Please label and include the following structures in your models.

1.) Hemagglutinin
2.) Membrane Protein
3.) Nucleocapsid

4.) RNA

## Spanish

**Essential Question**: How has the influenza virus affected the Spanish Culture. Discuss the history of the Spanish FLU 1918

Ask students what do they know about the flu?

Allow students to discuss the various things they may have heard in the media before showing a power point with information on the flu virus.
After the Power Point, allow students to create a bilingual information flyer or brochure.

The Brochure will have the following information concerning the Influenza Virus

5.) Brief History
6.) Symptoms
7.) Treatment
8.) How to Prevent the Spread of Influenza
One side of the Flyer or Brochure will be in English while the other side is in Spanish
All information on the CDC site can be translated into any language.

This curriculum allows students to see how each subject is important in delivering information in a way that relates to a current real-life scenario. Students began to understand and develop a better understanding of the basic history of a virus as well as preventive strategies needed to prevent the spread of disease.

# 12

# STEM 4 LIFE

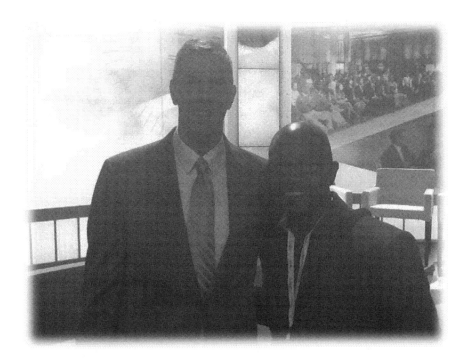

**Secretary of Education, Arnie Duncan and Evern Williams, MSNBC Education Summit 2012**

Attending several conferences allowed me to understand a more global insight of the epidemics across the world. I began developing

activities and curriculum that would bring awareness to these global epidemics to students. The National Science Foundation recognizes epidemiology as a STEM discipline.
https://www.lsamp.org/help/help_stem_cip_2010.cfm

Epidemiology can be taught with several disciplines within a unit. Although this article was produced in 2010, I was constantly reminded by professional learning institutions that Epidemiology did not fit into the subject area of STEM. Several either ignored the facts or did not have the time to see that public health was a great example STEM learning.

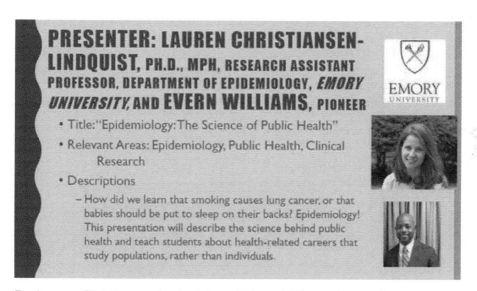


Dr. Lauren Christiansen-Lindquist, and Evern Williams Presenting to students in Gwinnett County Georgia, 2017

Real world application of math and science requires one to understand the idea and concept of curriculum integration. STEM an acronym for Science Technology Engineering and Math requires teachers from different disciplines to coordinate a curriculum lesson that utilizes each subject to solve a real-world scenario or problem. Will students learn more from what affect their lives? Is problem-based learning effective?

While teaching public health and epidemiology within the context of STEM and problem-based learning in a public-school system, I found it resourceful to categorize all the content for each subject into the five distinct frameworks. The students loved this method as it allowed them to easily recognize the relationship between all the topics.

The standards for science classes, STEM and Career Path standards are easily visible and are easily categorized when using the five frameworks of teaching Epidemiology and Public Health. This framework also identifies areas for integrating subjects and or cross cutting. The biggest setback of implementing these teaching strategies is trying to match them with your core curriculum, state standards and national standards. For example, there are the Georgia Standards for Excellence, National Science Teacher Standards and the Career Path to public Health standards. Teaching the class is one thing but making sure all standards are covered from the various levels seems to be a challenge for several educators. The problem-solving frameworks of History, Descriptive, Analytical, Ethical and Public Health Surveillance is a useful tool for designing cross cutting curricula and integrating different subjects. It allows students and educators to easily identify the various subject areas needed to solve real world problems. When teaching a global epidemic of water borne illness, I always provide students with the facts of the epidemic and allow them to divide the information up into the various categories. One of the most interesting global epidemics to me deaths due to water borne illnesses.

It is hard to believe that currently there is a global epidemic killing more than 2 million children each year. That is roughly 5, 479 children a day and more than 38,356 children a week. This epidemic affects those who are living in absolute poverty. Those experiencing absolute poverty struggle with the necessities of life. Food, clothing, shelter and clean available water has always been a struggle for those living under these conditions. As a result, an epidemic of deaths caused by water borne illnesses has emerged as one of the greatest killers of children within these countries. Water borne illnesses are infections caused by pathogens that are transmitted by consuming contaminated water. In 2010 the Centers for Disease Control and Prevention reported that the United States had a total of 1045 waterborne illnesses associated with drinking contaminated water. Out of the 1045 cases, only 85 were hospitalized with 9 deaths reported. In Africa alone more than 2.5 million children die each year because they do not have clean water to drink. That breaks down to more than 7,000 children per day, 47,000 children a week and 188,000 children each month. These numbers are probably astounding to most, but it is true and maybe a little bit low according to some numbers toping 3.6 million children deaths related to unsafe water worldwide.

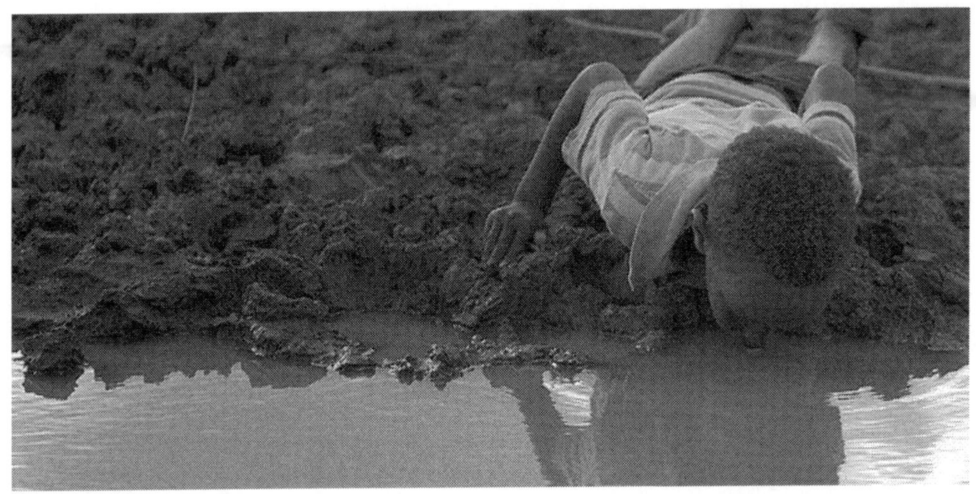

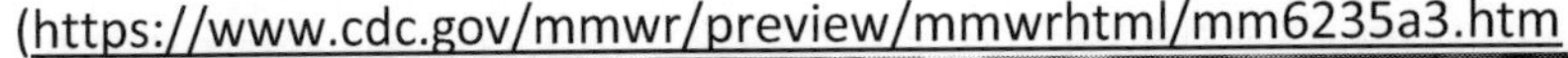

(https://www.cdc.gov/mmwr/preview/mmwrhtml/mm6235a3.htm

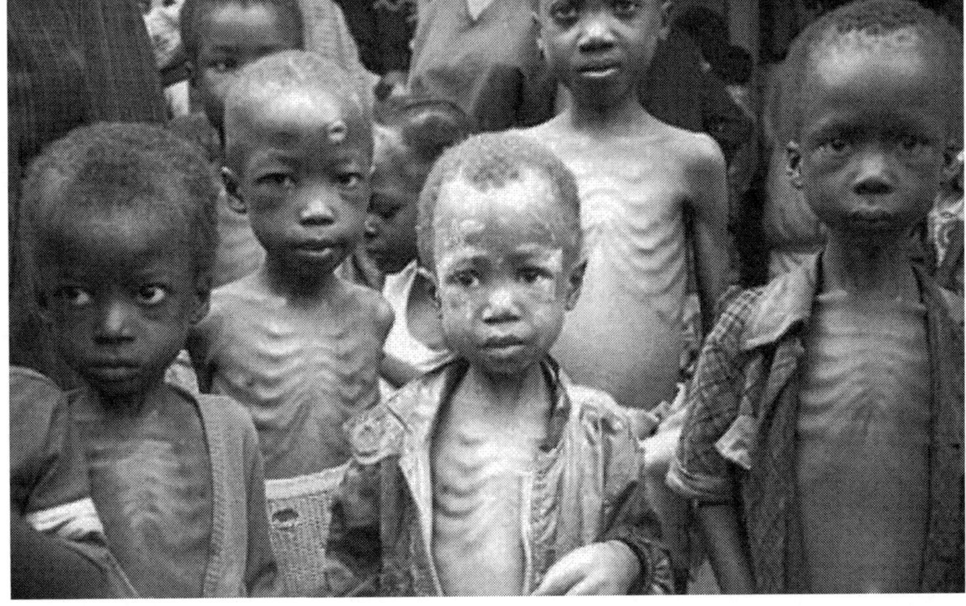

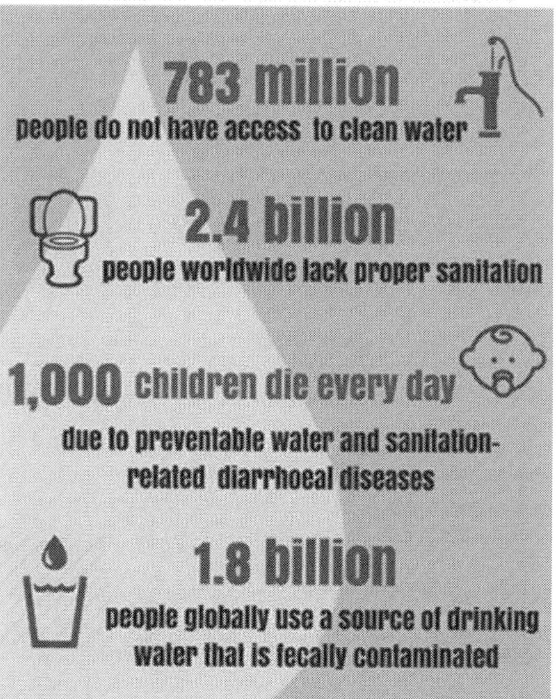

Water and Sanitation
783 million
people do not have access to clean water
2.4 billion
people worldwide lack proper sanitation
1,000 children die every day
due to preventable water and sanitation-related diarrhoeal diseases
1.8 billion
people globally use a source of drinking water that is fecally contaminated


The World Health Organization, WHO reports that there are more than 3.4 million deaths per year resulting from water borne diseases. This unit allows students the ability to learn understand and work on a project that is based on a global epidemic. This would work for a STEM class. This also allows students the ability to analyze, interpret, research and create new ideas and solutions. The problem is clearly identified in this unit. The idea of making and creating a solution or device that may provide clean water for the children is the objective. Students need to identify the cause and effect of the specific epidemic. Is it a virus, bacteria, protozoan, or worm? They will then create solutions to this problem by building a device that may serve as a filtering system for contaminated drinking water. Students can work individually or in teams. One could also enhance this activity by making it a competition. This lesson works well with students and or adults for professional training.

This lesson focuses on the ability of students understanding, analyzing summarizing and developing a product aimed at reducing the spread of waterborne illness. Instructors have the flexibility as to the depth of knowledge delivered to the class. After analyzing the data on this lesson students can research the common infections causing death within a specific region. Will developing a filtration device reduce the transmission rate of spreading the Guinea worm infection? Students can use critical thinking skills to analyze information and describe and produce a solution to this problem.

***Lesson Plan for filtration device***:

Teaching students how to build a filtration device for filtering microorganisms from contaminated water. Students will receive information and notes from the instructor on the epidemic of water borne illnesses internationally. I would begin the lesson with teaching students the History of water borne illness along with the types of microorganisms responsible for the deaths. We will also study the pathology of the microorganism and how it affects the human body. Students will then identify the characteristics of those affected from the epidemic, (Descriptive), person, place and time. They will research the data and geographical location of the epidemic. They will also analyze the specific subgroups mostly affected by the illness.

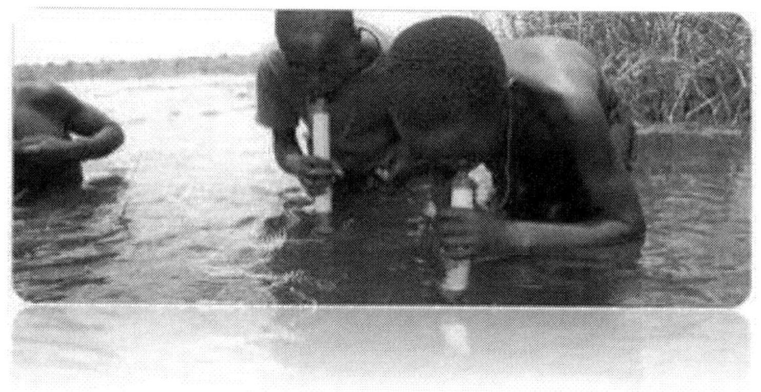

Lesson plan for filtration device activity:

The students will observe and learn of the ethical conditions that may affect this epidemic. Are there regulations for clean water and are there any laws and or policies that may prevent the development of such an underdeveloped country. Finally, students will begin to follow the scientific method in order to describe a solution. They will be coached into the mindset of an engineer given the task of creating a device that will filter the water for the children. The students may be divided into groups or pairs. I would not recommend for students working alone as within a normal environment engineers are more likely to work in groups or teams. It is at this point I would teach the scientific method as well as review STEM problem solving methods. The students will use the information from reviews, lectures and discussions gathered into the five frameworks and utilize this information to solve the problem.

They will begin to research filtration devices and the various natural resources that can be used to make a filtration device. Those in third world countries may have very few resources. The coach may want to guide the students to either restrict their materials to what is or may be available within the regions of those most affected by this epidemic. Or they can be given a set of material from the local hardware store and build a device effective for filtering these microorganisms.

PowerPoint, Lecture notes:
List of material one can use to make filtration device.
Material:

1. PVC pipes, pre cut. s
2. PVC Connectors/PVC cement optional
3. Charcoal Gravel, Sand
4. Mesh Screen material
5. Coffee Filters, Cups,
6. Water Analysis KIT / Optional

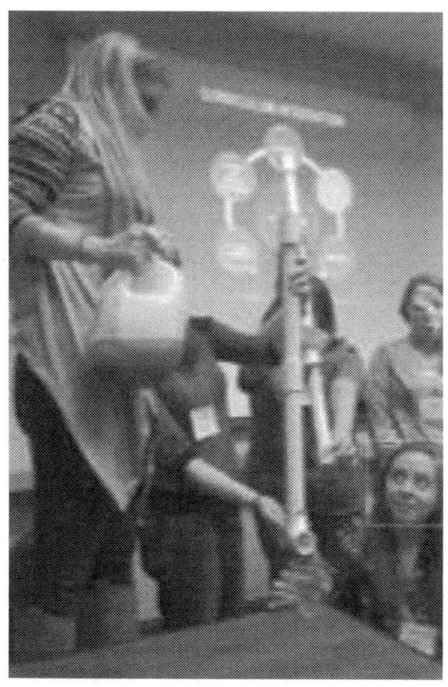

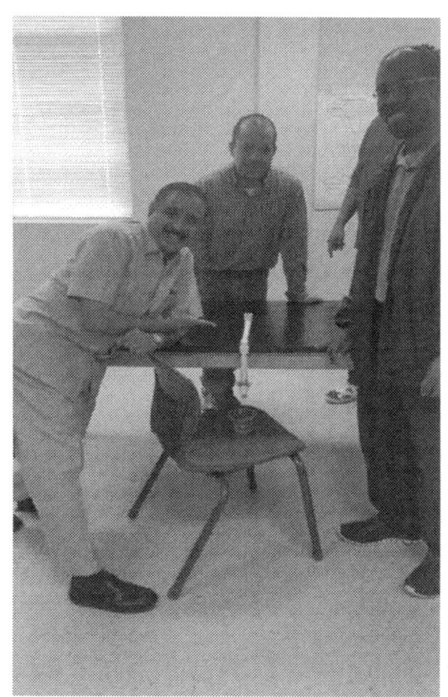

**Educators from District and State Conference build Filtration Devices for Competition**

# 13

# Environmental and Community Epidemics

Could Epidemiology help build positive relationships with teachers and students? Epidemiology allows teachers and students the ability to approach a topic in school from a growth mindset. How do you walk into a classroom and not have a plan for discussing a problem that 80% of your teenagers have discussed at home before entering the school building? How would a teacher begin to discuss the tragic events of the summer of 2016 with an extremely high number of police reported and recorded deaths of black males? Is it ethical to discuss the number of recent deaths caused by police officers during the summer of 2016? Is this something that can be discussed in a classroom? These questions rarely have direct answers. Is it ok then to discuss the influence of social media? "What about the epidemic of homicide within our communities". Can we discuss the fact that these events may not be an epidemic and merely a reflection of the amount of advanced technology within our society? Or is it best to ignore the student's comments and try to change the subject as they constantly try to engage teachers in conversations that may seem to make many uncomfortable? Maybe we live by subliminal rules that require us to never discuss specific topics until challenged. Or you could just say "I can't talk about that in class" like most teachers would probably say. Regardless, we cannot simply ignore the problems and challenges our children face each day within their own communities.

Community epidemics have a direct effect on the citizens who live within the affected areas. These epidemics range from infectious and chronic disease to addiction and mental illness. From bacterial and virus infections to opioid abuse and suicide. Allowing students to highly engage in real world problems in which they may have personal experiences could increase interest and awareness for community involvement. Beyond infectious diseases, there are behavioral and social epidemics that affect and strike hardest in poor and minority communities. The range of community epidemics are unlimited and may vary based on location and culture. These community problems directly affect the academic performance of our students each day. Although most may be familiar with associating epidemiology with only infectious diseases several of the community epidemics stretch far into the field of social epidemics. Poverty, Social Media Influence, homicide, bullying, drug addiction, suicide, human trafficking may all be considered social epidemics. Each of these topics can be taught in a public health and or epidemiology classroom. The same five frameworks are used to categorize the specific areas that will allow for students to accurately diagnose information regarding the subject or case study.

For any of the epidemic and public health topics students can perform community projects and create solutions as they follow the frameworks. These topics may provide a more interesting, exciting and relevant curriculum. A curriculum that relates to the world from which they live. Our student can go back and speak to their family members and peers about public health issues they find interesting. They may also inspire others to go out and get involved in community projects.

Number of leading causes of death in the United States.
www.cdc.gov/nchs/fastats/leading-causes-of-death.htm

- Heart disease: 647,457
- Cancer: 599,108
- Accidents (unintentional injuries): 169,936
- Chronic lower respiratory diseases: 160,201
- Stroke (cerebrovascular diseases): 146,383
- Alzheimer's disease: 121,404
- Diabetes: 83,564
- Overdose Deaths: 67,000
- Influenza and Pneumonia: 55,672
- Nephritis, nephrotic syndrome and nephrosis: 50,633
- Intentional self-harm (suicide): 47,173

How can we teach such a sensitive topic in a class filled with policies, procedures and laws that prevent educators from discussing these relevant subjects? When discussing statistical analysis of current epidemics for subgroups we are then given the opportunity to teach a topic that may be sensitive yet informative and relevant. This allows the instructor to introduce a topic and engage group discussions based on data. In my experiences it is always important to lead sensitive topics by discussing its relevance based on statistics before getting into any discussions. It is within this chapter that I briefly describe some of the most recent and relevant community epidemics that a large majority of the population may have experienced. Some in which you may not think of as an epidemic, however anything that is considered a health threat and shows a significant increase over time can possibly be considered an epidemic.

**Poverty Epidemic**.

Today our students face various challenges that may hinder their interest from reading at all. Several subgroups fall behind as they may lose interest in academics due to more challenging problems and circumstances. A large segment of our society does not have equal opportunities as others based on their culture, immediate family surroundings and or socioeconomic position. Can we teach students the epidemic of poverty in the classroom? Will it be useful for them and their future? The epidemic of poverty and other community problems are topics that can teach students preventive strategies that may assist them in avoiding negative revolving ties to old family values.

For years children of lower socioeconomic subgroups have demonstrated less interest in education, lower test scores and higher dropout rates. Either they decide to give in to the peer pressures around them or fall directly into the stereotypes generated by the media, immediate family or neighborhood friends. Others may decide to make a bad decision since they do not know any other way. If this is true, is there a way to teach students how to make better decisions and think about their every action and how it affects others. Discussing the epidemic of poverty allows students the opportunity to work on problem solving strategies that may help them break the chains of poverty within their own family.

Children who suffers from poverty have less opportunities of within the middle and upper classes. Several of these students may have less experience with cultural, and social opportunities based on financial income. They may need to eat what they have available and not what is best for them to maintain good health. Poor diet with a lack of adequate grocery stores within these neighborhoods have led to a community of people with increased health risks. With the lack of transportation several may never get the opportunity to visit a grocery store for days. Common gas stations and convenient stores have made their way to most corner stores and may commonly sale basic items of grocery and snacks replace healthy fruits and vegetables. What happens when a student is provided two honey buns and a Juice for breakfast and had nothing to eat for dinner. Assume this is a 9-year-old young man approaching school full of sugar and excitement from the smell of a hot breakfast. The student's future is in the hands of those who teach them. A misdiagnosis of mental illness is crucial to the student's future. hype. He or she may be encouraged to see a psychologist and given a prescription for some form of mental illness that may not exist. Is it possible for anyone to get a misdiagnosis for mental illness? Have we made it too easy to label our children with mental illnesses and provide them with psychological medicines that may have unknown long-term effects? This could easily be a systemic issue that encourages misdiagnosis of young black males in elementary schools.

Not only does students in poverty struggle with poor diet and health, but they may also suffer with more mental illness and peer pressure from conditions of social and financial status. The electricity may get cut off; they may have to move to different area after being evicted. They may suffer from a lack of supplies and access to technology at home to complete homework assignments. Computers, smartphones, iPad, or androids are just a few of the items that a child living in poverty may not have available. May not feel comfortable attending school at times because of clothing conditions, or cleaning ability. If there is no water, they may not be able to shower properly and select to stay at home rather than deal with the embarrassment and shame. As a result, they may make the choice to skip school for a few days until their home situation gets better. Poverty has always created a wedge in the education of our youth. A topic that can be discussed and diagnosed with students and adults beyond the boundaries of school walls reaching all those within the communities. While serving as a prevention intervention specialist in Newton County, our Deputy Superintendent pursued and introduced poverty training for our entire district. I attended a poverty training workshop that introduced poverty as something that must be understood by educators in order to see the needs of all our children.

While teaching the ethics of the epidemic of poverty I have learned to understand the effects of systemic barriers that retain those in poverty making it almost difficult to escape their reality. I have had my own experiences with poverty both in real life and during a professional learning class. During part of a poverty training we were sent into the community dressed in old or dirty clothing. We were given the task of going out to look for assistance from a variety of places and companies set up to assist those who were looking for food, clothing, shelter, and financial assistance or work. Our group went to a local weekly hotel looking for a place to sleep for one night. I went there with two of my colleagues and was received astonishing results in our experience trying to get a room. One of my colleagues was white he and I are about the same age. He went in and asked for a room and was informed that they had two rooms left and was given a price of 165.00 a week. The receptionist for the hotel did not know we were in the same vehicle. I eventually got out of the vehicle and went inside to ask for a room. The receptionist gave me a price of 185.00 a week and informed me that they did not have any rooms available. My colleague looked at me with disbelief. Yet he could not say a word as we did not want the receptionist to know we were on a scavenger hunt for support. We discussed this with the entire district upon our return. We reported to the group that I possessed a double edge sword in my appearance in my pursuit of happiness. I was identified as a poor black man. A big difference from being a poor person of any other race as a man. My colleagues were surprised that I was treated with such harsh, rude and uncaring employees that are employed to provide services for those in need. It is an experience that in fact most people of poverty deal with each day. One can only imagine what some people must deal with as adults and to make matters worse, you have a teenager watching you struggle throughout it all. Providing students an avenue to have an outlet of open discussion in the classroom may help build a bridge of support between children in need and the school system.

## Social Media Influence

When I was young my mother would hold my hand as I walked beside her. This was her way of protecting me from strangers, kidnappers and other violent criminals. The rapid rise of the internet has allowed students access to a world of information and people. The advancements of science and technology has allowed students access to an entire world at their fingertips. Current issues in the news, and social media can be seen by students in a matter of seconds from around the world. Every day we see a current issue on television, or social media. Everyday students get an opportunity to bring this topic into the classroom for discussion. A really easy way to bring real world application into any curriculum.

Currently, our society is filled with criminals who are master manipulators using technology as the tool of choice. Children are not always communicating with a neighbor or close relative when upset. Some would say that the technology age has led to the information age. At the click of a button children, teenagers and adults can access information with limitless boundaries in a matter of seconds. As a result, our children and or young adults are exposed to unlimited amounts of information from the internet nevertheless, all the information they retrieve may be meet with manipulation and negative intentions.

Our students may benefit from learning the epidemic of social media influence. There are pros and cons to every situation. Although social media has its negative drawbacks it does serve as an efficient resource for everyone if used in a positive way. The world is at your fingertips with a click of a button. Media influence is important when it comes to obtaining customers for business minded entrepreneurs and those with extraordinary talents and gifts. Several recent overnight success entertainers started out on social media. Our current political leaders continue to battle for media approval and influence. They are aware of the influence it has on the human mind and is often used to campaign and influence decisions before elections. They too have begun to understand the power of social media and the amount of influence it has over all Americans.

Over the past ten years I think we can all agree how we have seen the influence of social media as a huge epidemic that may affect other epidemics. Challenges, both safe and dangerous have surged over social media. Suicides and bullying have become another epidemic that may have been encouraged by social media. How can we begin a discussion on the social media epidemic and how it has influenced other epidemics?

The skills learned from a public health and epidemiology class allows students the opportunity to discuss and include such current issues within the classroom and curriculum. They understand where to obtain accurate information and can determine if information is relevant or not. The opportunity to discuss how social media influence our lives allows some students who may have been victims an outlet. Educators can discuss and deliver programs, hotlines, and social organizations that may assist a student during a crisis or abuse.

For most teenager's social media is used more for entertainment rather than educational purposes. Is the internet safe or does it provide a new way to lure teenagers into a web of deception? We must begin to have these discussions with our students as the world we live in has changed and become much larger than the communities we live within.

Engaging students in activities and topics that demonstrate how the media influence our decisions is a topic that most children and teenagers can relate. Today, most children and teenagers are glued to their phones. Their either watching YouTube, snapchat or some other form of social media communication. Students have even discovered that one can get famous based on the number of views or subscriptions one may have on their channel. Encouraging students to utilize social media as a tool for projects gives them the opportunity to utilize their device for learning. An Epi project may include surveys designed to document common reasons for social media use. I am sure administrators have seen an increase of social media as the cause of conflicts among students. Not only is it an issue for students but for adults as well. Imagine being an educator and your mugshot appears on social media. You are suddenly the talk of the entire town. How does an educator prepare for this moment? Are there any ethical guidelines that may provide protocol for such an event? Or how does social media exploit you when a company offers to help you with your reputation by taking it down for $700.00 dollars. Yes, I was that teacher. I got arrested and got a mugshot or two go up for unfortunate circumstances. I had to deal with it head on and discuss the importance of maintaining calmness even when you think or know your right.

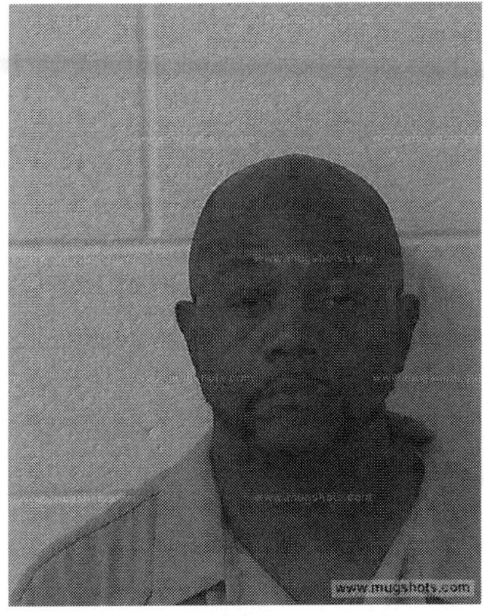


I knew there was a mistake or something, however, I was a black man being asked to get out the car by the police and put my hands behind my back. I followed the instructions and based on recent videos surfacing pertaining to black men and police, I am thankful that I had officers who were truly professional. Once again, I have always been trained by my mother to not argue or cause a disruption with a police officer.

The students respected my unfortunate experience and understood how sometimes things will go bad even when you think you are doing right. It is how you react in the moment that determines whether you survive the storm. I remember the last time I was arrested in Covington, GA during the spring of 2016, I was in a holding cell with some of my former students. They shared their misfortunes with me and why they were in the position they were in. I did not respond in any different manner than if they were in my classroom. I let them know their risky behavior patterns may lead to a life of long-term prison time or death. Even though this was a rough situation for me to be in, I did not change who I was to them while I was in the cell. I was still Mr. Williams, just sitting behind bars. I had to keep pushing. Regardless of my circumstances I was determined to continue moving forward.

Over the summer of 2016 several young black men were killed by officers on duty. Some were even recorded live on social media during the killing. Several were outraged and utilized social media as an outlet to express feelings. Social Media brings awareness to information that may not make the news. Black Lives Matter began as a slogan for racial injustice and developed into a movement for social justice and reform. All lives matter is now a statement showing an opposition to Black Lives Matter. All the ethical parameters were set by social media. I was recently corrected and had to get an understanding myself of why anyone may personally feel that all lives matter, the statement is to remind all the world and America that black lives matter. Social media controlled the entire movement which spread across the world. This is a clear example of how social media has influenced our lives and even behaviors.

Employers use social media to view the lifestyle of the person they are hiring while some companies continue to monitor and view social media post of their employees to ensure they are ethically and morally able to represent the company. Over the past 10 years hundreds of state, and local employees lost jobs due to unethical postings on social media. With the increase of social media platforms, our society has an outlet for everyone from all different ages and cultures

Students may engage in projects that involve positive social media platforms for positive community outcomes. And to assist as mentees to several community assistance programs and volunteer for activities.

In 2017 my epidemiology students from Newton High School decided to assist in promoting and supporting a community fun run for a local drug prevention and addiction rehabilitation company. They participated and voluntarily promoted a 5k fun run to assist those suffering from drug addiction. Although the moment was exhausting, it was well worth the experience and joy seen on their faces while running. I caught with a few of them during the run and talked about their experiences. They were glad to be a part of something big and for a positive cause within their own community. When teaching of public health and epidemiology students can experience a world beyond the classroom.

Picture of fun run.

## Cocaine and Crack epidemic

Community epidemics are an ever-increasing problem that affect student performance. Some of the most common of these epidemics are those that may be caused from social economic issues. When looking at each of these topics we must understand and ask ourselves the question. What do all these topics have in common? They all affect the human population with statistical data analysis of studies to be considered an epidemic because the numbers have increased over the years. It is a common mathematical denominator of biostatistics. Since 1947 the CDC began the quest of developing the science of epidemiology and public health. Any disease, social action, or other phenomena that causes an increase in deaths from year to year should be considered an epidemic. Currently when I began to think of the most common epidemics that affect our community several may come to mind. For years there have been several communities from rural and urban cities plagued by public health issues affecting health, socioeconomic, federal aid, and death rates for specific subgroups. As an African American male, I can certainly relate to the epidemics that affect our communities and lives. However, I have noticed that these epidemics have changed over the years. In the early 1980's crack began to rise as the drug of choice in neighborhoods of minority communities. This was the beginning of a major drug epidemic that devastated communities and families throughout the nation. The history of this epidemic began in the early to mid-1980's. In the 70's the drug of choice was heroine which was later replaced by cocaine both consumed by injection or snorting through the nostrils. Cocaine was once associated with financially successful individuals while crack cocaine was more associated with those of a lower economic class. Crack is cocaine mixed with a base and smoked instead of being snorted in its original form. The price of crack cocaine was substantially cheaper than cocaine therefore it was a drug of choice for those in low income areas. Costing as little as 5 to 10 or 20 dollars made it the drug of choice for those living in low socioeconomic communities which were primarily those communities of color. Crack cocaine also influenced the spread of other epidemics such as HIV, Human Immunodeficiency virus, gonorrhea and herpes. As a result, HIV began to increase as the crack epidemic increased. Descriptive epidemiology describes person, place and time. Who was affected by crack? When did this occur? And in what cities or communities did this epidemic begin to thrive? These are some of the questions we must begin to talk about with our students. Epidemiology teaches students how to follow trends using real world data. Although the crack epidemic began in the 1980's we can teach it as a part of the history of how drug epidemics affect our communities. It is hard for students to understand how to find a solution to a problem if you do not truly know the history of the problem. The project may consider discussing the most recent drug epidemic which are methamphetamines, pentenyl, heroine and prescription opiate abuse. Students may present projects of awareness and possible solutions to the problems sent as a suggestion for policy changes. Or at the least bring attention and awareness to some of the community programs available within their own community.

.

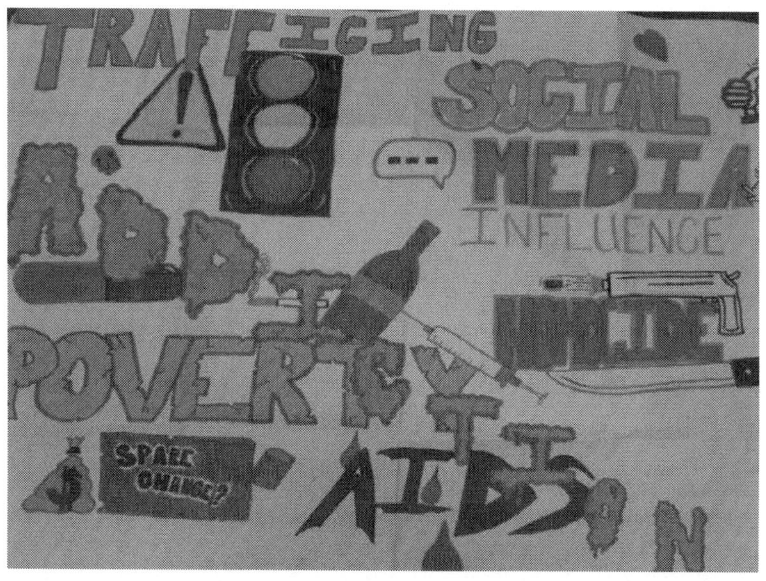


**Example of Student Artwork Reflecting Community Epidemics**

## Suicide and Opioid Addiction

A recent journal from the National Science Journal of Health identified that this is the first time that the life expectancy for humans have dropped since 1993. Primarily due to two disturbing epidemics. Suicide and opioid addiction both very epidemics that affect communities and families.

https://www.hhs.gov/blog/2017/04/03/public-health-crisis-suicide-and-opioids.html.

Counselors, teachers, students, and parents may all benefit from understanding how these epidemics may affect them and their community. I think we can all say that addiction is certainly a real-world issue that is relevant to all people. We must educate students parents and the community on such topics. Suicide was the cause of more than 44,500 deaths in 2015 and almost 70,000 in 2017 according to the CDC. One of the greatest contributors of the suicide epidemic is the ever-growing trend of drug abuse in the United States. Synthetic fentanyl, heroine, and prescribed opioid abuse are some of the most devasting drugs destroying both minority and majority communities. All have been linked to deaths by abuse and overdoses. Today we have commercials on television that clearly describes one or more of the long-term effects is giving you thoughts of suicide. This is known in the public health world as a side effect of a drug. Our students hear the messages and have learned to interpret information as either fact or fiction. Ethics of epidemiology allows students to see how certain policies and laws affect an epidemic. Students can once again understand Cause and Effect as it relates to public health. Along with prescription meds, offering side effects of suicide other illegal drugs from the past have made their way back into our communities. Prescription opioids, heroine, methamphetamines, and synthetic fentanyl are responsible for more than 70,000 deaths in 2017 according to the National Center for Health Statistics at the Centers for Disease Control and Prevention.

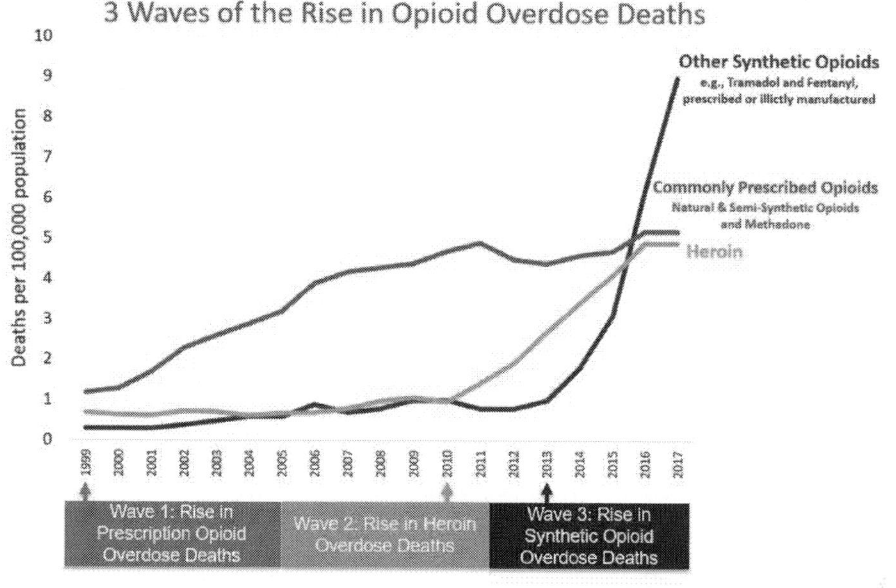


https://www.cdc.gov/drugoverdose/images/epidemic/3WavesOfTheRiseInOpioidOverdoseDeaths.png

Figure 4. **National Drug Overdose Deaths Involving Prescription Opioids,** Number Among All Ages, 1999-2017

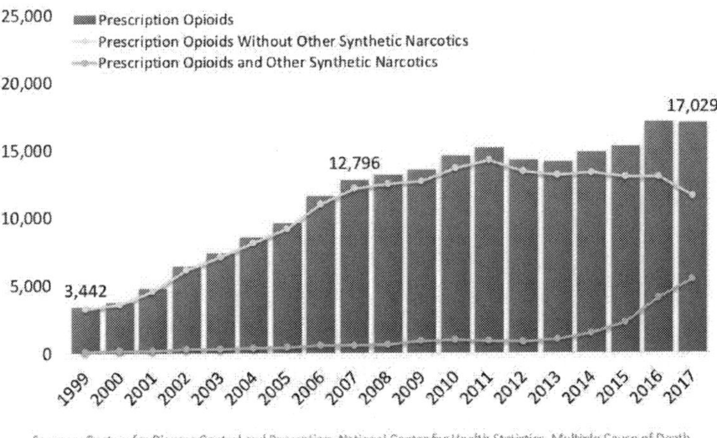


Source: : Centers for Disease Control and Prevention, National Center for Health Statistics. Multiple Cause of Death 1999-2017 on CDC WONDER Online Database, released December, 2018

Figure 1. **National Drug Overdose Deaths** Number Among All Ages, by Gender, 1999-2017

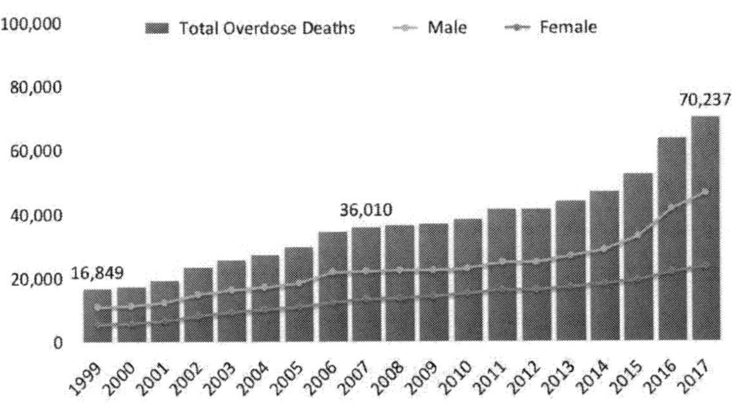


Source: : Centers for Disease Control and Prevention, National Center for Health Statistics. Multiple Cause of Death 1999-2017 on CDC WONDER Online Database, released December, 2018

Opioid addiction is one of the fastest growing addictions within the community over the last ten years. At one point in our lives we would only hear of famous people suffering from prescription drug addiction. Yet over the past 15 years it has become a wrecking ball within all communities affecting all ages races and income levels. How does the addiction epidemic affect a community? Almost every student from middle school and above either knows someone or is related to an individual fighting some type of drug addiction. Since prescription opioids and heroin are made from the poppy plant, it should not surprise anyone of the growing number of consumers addicted to prescription pain pills. These and other addictions may lead to financial and social destruction of both families and communities. Crime is likely to follow addiction in some cases to support their habit. The number of people affected by the side effects of addiction are far greater than the addiction statistics. Epidemics such as suicides, incarceration rates, poverty, homicides, and the number of single parent homes are all affected by addiction. Drug overdose deaths increased from 38,000 in 2010 to 70,000 in 2017.

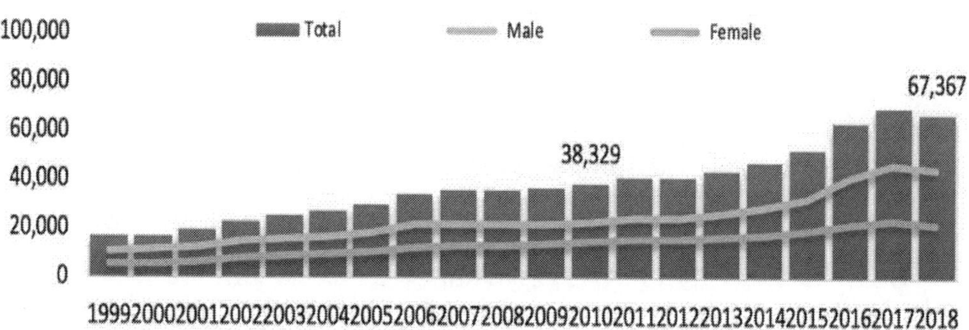

For all of those reading this book thinking that tomorrow is not worth pushing forward. I can only tell you what works for me when life seems to just throw you that curve ball called obstacle. No matter how hard it gets remember that tomorrow is another day. Depression is alive and well within our population. It is a mood disorder which causes someone to become sad, lose interest, and withdraw from others. About one in 15 Americans may suffer from depression. I personally experienced a depressive state within my own life.

Before the 2009-2010 school year I was informed that I had to resign as a teacher because there were no proof of any of my professional learning units on file. I was forced to resign and accept substitute pay. I was deeply depressed and stunned beyond belief. To lose your teaching certificate and job after teaching for nearly 14 years was like a sickness I carried in my stomach for months. A hard pill to swallow every day. I went from teacher to substitute overnight. It was like a living nightmare. One that I could not believe was happening. Imagine teaching in your profession for 13 years with all certifications and qualifications. Your told you could only be utilized as a substitute teacher doing the same job for one third of the pay. I had no choice but to take the substitute pay. We were in a recession in 2009 as there were very few jobs available within our community. I taught the physical science classes as a substitute teacher while working with the CDC to obtain my professional learning units. After a few months as a sub I obtained enough professional learning units to get my certification back and was then informed by the district that I could not get my job as a teacher back.

The reason is that they were not hiring any more teachers after February for the school year. I went into a spiral of depression and sadness.

. Engulfed in deep depression and sadness I had to take some type of control of my life and put energy in a different direction. Knowing at the time that mental illness and suicide deaths were increasing every year, I was determined not to allow current circumstances to control my entire life. I felt as if I was being oppressed for being an educated black man. I wanted to get away from everyone, I withdrew from those that were close to me.

As a result, I decided to take myself on a trip to New York city for my 40th birthday. On a budget and seeking a mental break I researched the National Action Network company. The conference featured speakers from all over the U.S. and celebrated education. It was truly a relaxing break for me trying to bounce back from sinking into depression. Although the conference was quite informative everyone wanted to go to the main banquet dinner attended by several big names and celebrities. I had only 60 dollars cash in my pocket. Certainly not enough to pay for a five-hundred-dollar ticket. However, I showed up and began mingling with the celebrities wearing one of my old polyester bell bottom suits with my conference badge. Without revealing how I got into the front of the stage with the celebrities. I will say that knowing music and being able to speak the language of music can go a long way when you are talking to talented musicians. I somehow found myself sitting at the very front of the banqueted event. After I looked around, I knew I had to be sitting in the VIP section as Mariah Carey and Nick Cannon were right in front of me while Regina King, Wyclef Jones and Bill Cosby were at the same table I was sitting.

After the event, all of those in the VIP section turned to one another and began to meet and greet. As I stood up Mariah turned around and as I reached to introduce myself Nick Cannon grabbed her shoulder and pulled her away. I think Regina King saw it. Or maybe she did not. I turned and began to communicate with her and decided to get a nice photo. I also meet other celebrities, and executives in various fields. No matter how bad things get you are only one day away from making it great. Never Stop pushing!

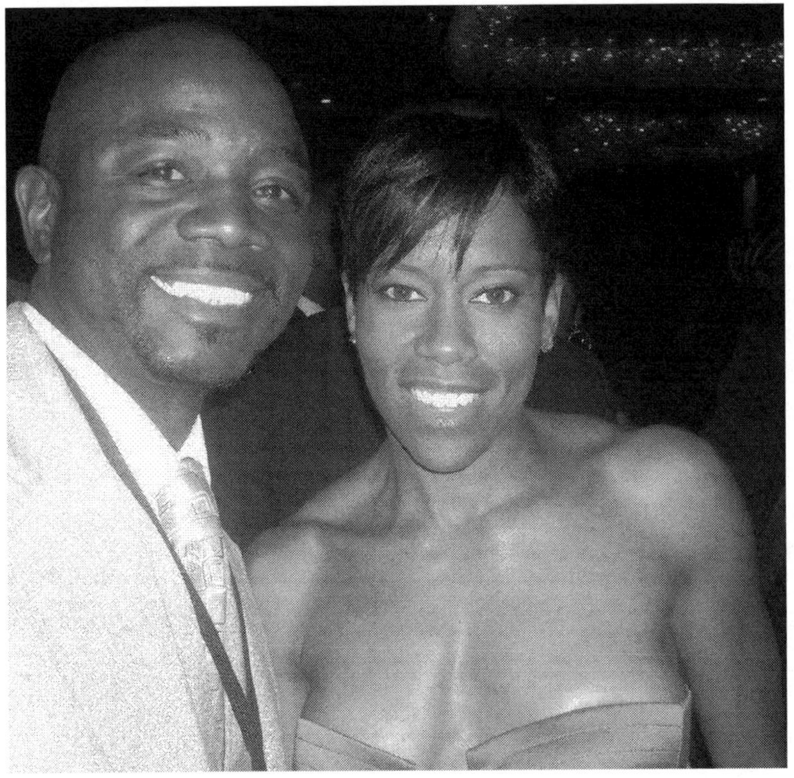

Regina King and Evern Williams NAN Conference Banquet 2010

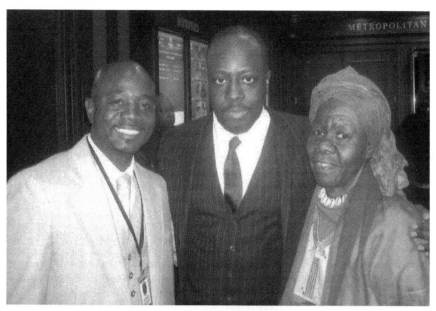


**Evern Williams and Wycleff 2010 NAN Conference**

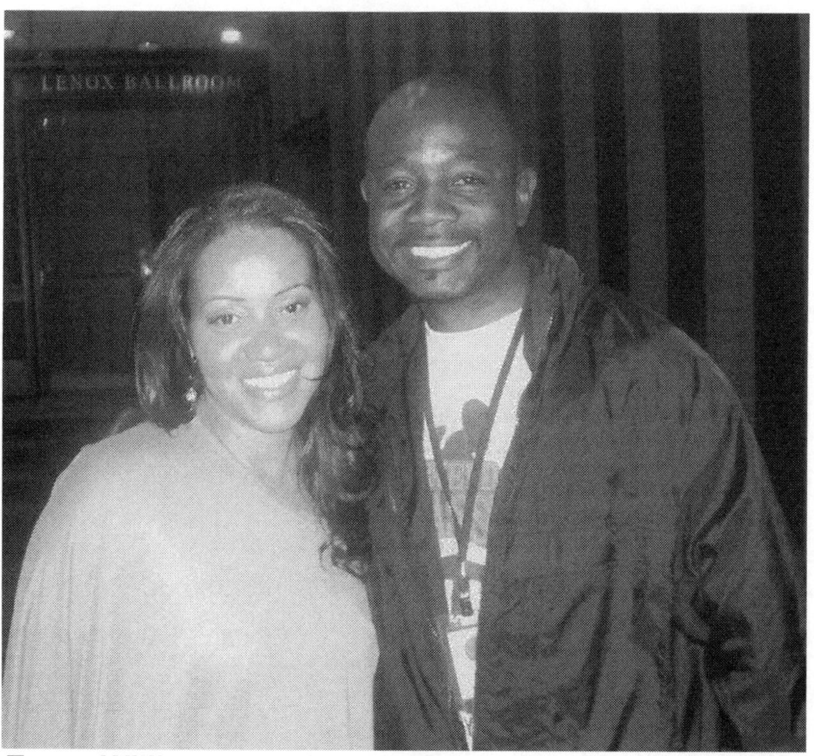


**Evern Williams and Cheryl "Salt" James NAN Conference 2010**

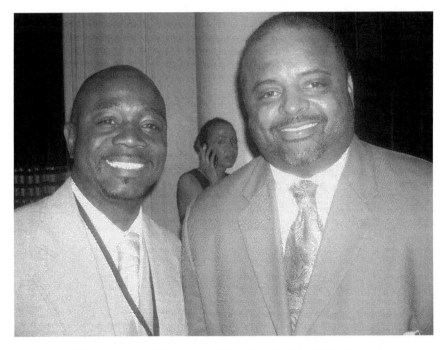

**Evern Williams and Roland Martin 2010 NAN Conference**

Shortly after returning from the trip to New York I received an email requesting my assistance with designing the framework for the first High School Epidemiology Class in the U.S. by state and federal organizations. I followed my purpose and continued to strive for the highest despite my obstacle. I Decided to not allow my situation to control my circumstances. Being forced to resign and take substitute pay until I paid for 100 hours led me back to the CDC. Never allow any situation to turn you from your purpose. I always say when you think you are at a dead end, think of it as a cul-de-sac for knowledge. I thank GOD for giving me the strength to endure it all.

Although I was strong enough mentally to pull myself out of a depressed state of mind, several are unable to overcome their own trials. They stay to themselves and fall deeper into depression. I urge all to reach out to those suffering from mental illness and depression as your communication just may be the key to saving a life.

**Homicide**

Homicide is another epidemic that affects all American communities. African American men between the age of 15 and 24 years of age are more likely to die by gunshot than any other way of death. Walking into a classroom and telling your class "The likely hood of everyone dying in this room is by suicide, unless you are an African American male between the ages of 15 and 24 years of age your likelihood of death would be by gunshot". The classroom gets silent and their eyes begin to look around as if I have said something that was wrong. Yet I began to show them the statistics of deaths in the United States along with the most affected subgroups from these specific epidemics. Allowing statistical data to lead the discussion on epidemics takes the pressure off the teacher, trainer and or instructor as it relies on numbers instead of personal opinions. The number of mass murders have increased over the past decade. As we are familiar with several mass murders at airports, places of employment, streets, night clubs and even schools within our communities. I remember teaching my epidemiology class after the Sandy Cook shooting and began looking for data on the number of deaths by gun violence and could not find anything. I contacted someone I knew who worked at the CDC and asked where to find the data on deaths caused by gun violence in the U.S. I was told that there was a policy in place that restricted the CDC from releasing any data on the number of gun violence caused deaths in the U.S. by lawmakers. A policy that was controlled by the National Rifle Association. Two years later, Obama ordered the release of this information following the Sandy Cook shooting. In a recent article titled"

"Elevated Rates of Urban Firearm Violence and Opportunities for Prevention" Despite a 2013 Executive order by President Barack Obama to resume research on gun violence, the CDC has adhered to a two-decade-old Congressional restriction that effectively bans such inquiries.
https://dhss.delaware.gov/dhss/dms/files/cdcgunviolencereport10315.pdf

Gathering data will involve history, descriptive and analytical information in order to guide your experiment. Ethical epidemiology covers the depth of your experiment including laws, culture, religion, and policies that may guide experimental studies to ensure legal practice. The experiment will be a part of the public health surveillance in which a student begins to test his or her experiment in order to find a possible solution. Whether or not the experiment may be deemed as a solution there must be a significant change in the data. For example. How can we decrease the number of black males from killing one another within the community? Students can all follow the framework, however each of them may want to focus on different variables that affect the outcome of numbers.

Recent project results from student project for possible solutions for improving relationships between officers and citizens.

Possible solutions:

1. Anti-Violence Seminars within communities with high crime rates
2. More small businesses within the community.
3. More affordable educational programs.
4. Training for all public workers especially police officers, Cultural Awareness Class, Cultural Identity
5. Teaching Young adults proper communication skills.
6. Media Influence awareness classes
7. Anti-bullying-Workplace-Bullying classes
8. De Escalation Classes for both police and citizens

Although the students did not get to test their solutions, they did get an opportunity to collaborate and create a proposed set of solutions. That can be measured in an assessment. If time permits, students can then test their experiment by implementing these projects within their school and or community.

The diagrams below symbolize how one epidemic may influence other epidemics. Does Addictions lead to mental illness and chemical dependency? Do those in poverty have a greater chance of being incarcerated or addicted by drugs. Does Systemic barriers affect those in poverty and prevent them from moving forward. How does a student who has no food and lights at home function at the same level as a student who eats three square meals a day and all the latest technology? Could stress and peer pressure lead to an addiction and or mental illness? I am sure that we may not have the answers to all the questions now but understanding that they do exist gives us the opportunity to begin to think of solutions.

Understanding every variable within a community problem, gives citizens and community leaders a better opportunity to create solutions with substance.

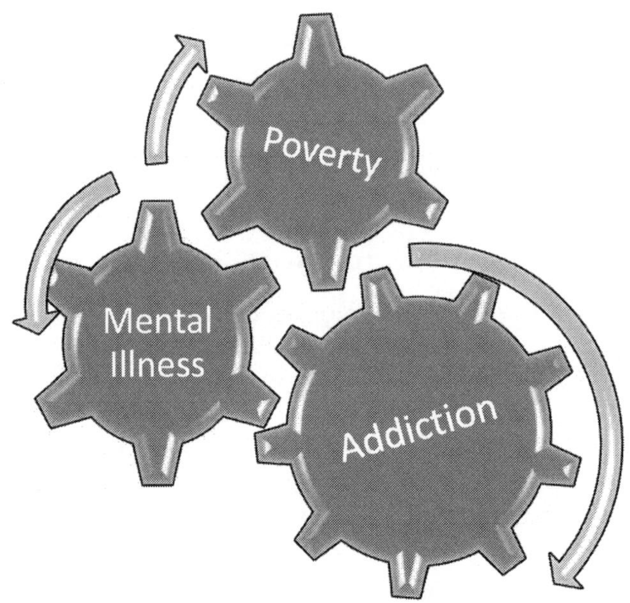


.

http://drugenquirer.com/side_effects/cfr/cfr_schedule2.html

**Mental Illness**

According to the National Institute of Mental Health, NIMH, one in five adults in the United States suffer from a mental illness. More than 47 Million adult Americans suffer with either a severe or any mental Illness. While growing up in the 70's and 80's the word mental illness was rarely heard especially within a school building. Now it is one of the most common discussions regarding student behavior. The National Ambulatory reported more than 58 million transports by ambulance were for diagnosed mental illness issues. While we continue to see a steady increase in the number of mental health patience, we may be increasing the gates to mental illness by increased intake with increased screenings. Is it possible for us to misdiagnose student in poverty for having a mental illness only because they had access to a honey bun and fruit punch for breakfast and dinner? In this scenario, the sugar breakfast now turns into a behavior uncontrolled problem that may spiral into a series of psychotic meds that the student may not need. What are the true long-term effects of consuming psychotic medication from the age of 8 to 18? Are we keeping up with the data within the different subgroups? Analyzing the data on mental illness cases along with subgroups enables one to begin to identify who the epidemic affects and why are they being affected.

According to some researchers, Ritalin, a common drug used to treat ADHD, attention deficit hyperactive disorder, has side effects that resembles that of cocaine and methamphetamine addiction. Those taking Ritalin may suffer from psychosis, nervousness, agitation, nausea and addiction.
http://www.rxlist.com/ritalin-side-effects-drug-center.htm

Will the surge to identify students suffering from mental illness lead to an increase in the epidemic of psychosis, schizophrenia or addiction ten years down the road? Mental illness affects those of all ages and races. Several may even suffer from a mental illness and not even know it and never get diagnosed.

Over the past 10 years another epidemic has affected Americans of all ages and races Mass shootings is an epidemic that affects all people, primarily targeting those who are defenseless and innocent. From airports to school buildings this problem does not discriminate and can cause several long-term effects for both victims and to those watching these violent acts. During my 24 years of teaching, several mass shootings have targeted public and private schools across the nation. Columbine High School, Newton Elementary School, Sandy Hook, Heritage High School, and the more recent Parkland Florida. Although we make a valid effort of preparing our students and staff for such an event, no one knows how an intruder with a semiautomatic rifle entering a building with the purpose of shooting anyone will affect an entire body of people until it happens. Over the past five years we have had more mass shootings than the last 50 years combined. Is there a correlation between mass shootings and mental illness? Currently both law makers and politicians are pushing the idea to keep guns out of the hands of those with a record of mental illness. Assuming most people committing such crimes have a mental illness they have already began the push to make changes to policies restricting those with a record of mental illness from purchasing weapons. No one has a specific answer to the problem or a solution to this horrific epidemic. As I witnessed my own students protest for the Parkland Florida shooting by walking out of class. I asked myself the question, “What am I going to say to them when they walk back into my classroom from the protest outside”? What are the liabilities of discussing this issue in a classroom? How do we begin to discuss the issue? Or is it ok to talk about this topic with your students? Teaching the five frameworks allows students the opportunity to discuss the pros and cons of such solutions. I did ask them after coming back into the room, “why did all of you go outside"? Most replied, "to support safe schools". Others said because "everybody knew to go outside because it's all over social media". From there our Epidemiology students began a discussion on the power of social media today.

Students recently discussed what they thought would make for a good solution for mass shootings in schools? They compare some of their ideas to those they have heard from political leaders. I will say that some of the past ideas such as allowing teachers to carry weapons and teaching them to defend themselves and students during a mass shooting may not be the safest method. What happens when one of the educators carrying a weapon has an undiagnosed mental illness and feels threated by a large male? Another problem! There could be multiple incidents of senseless crimes for allowing teachers to carry guns in schools. Using the frameworks allows students to diagnose this problem and help create a possible solution.

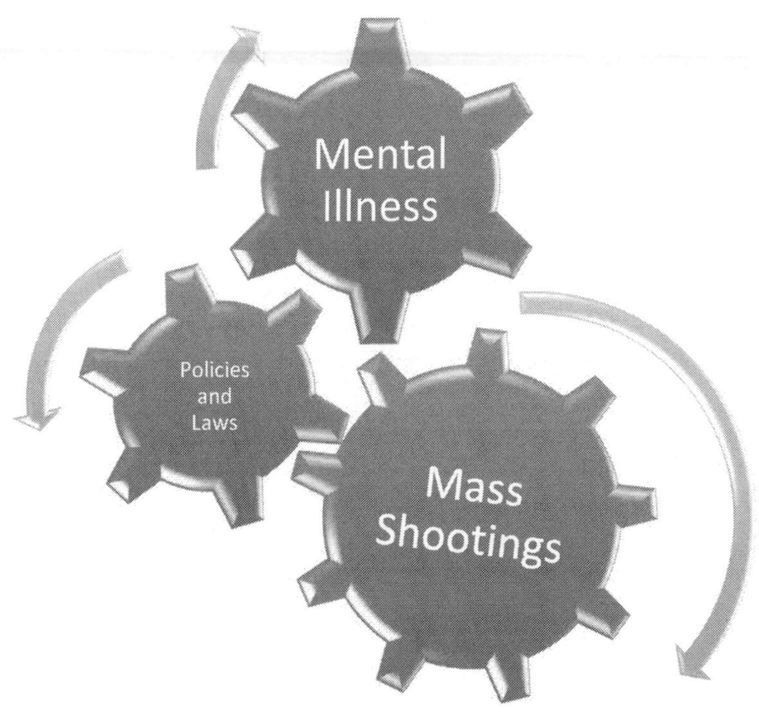


**Mass Incarceration of African American Males**

Mass incarceration rate of African American males in the United States is one of the most unbalanced epidemics based on culture. African American males make up about 6% of the population yet it makes up more than 70% of the prison population. Why is there a greater chance for African American males to go to prison instead of college? Or why does statistics show that one in every three black men will go to prison or jail while one in 10 black men will attend college. Does the media in America portray black males in a negative light? I have heard opinions on both sides. Yet one thing is true based on history of entertainment and black males. Black males have been portrayed as wild savages since the very first movie filmed in America, "Birth of a Nation". In this Movie, black males were viewed and depicted as savages and the KKK would come to save the day. With the advancement from television to social media several entrepreneurs have taken this opportunity to show other sides of issues affecting black males.

In a classroom an instructor would follow the framework and begin with the direct correlation to the numerical data. One out of every three males going to prison is thirty percent (30%). This is an example of a description epidemiology identifying person, place and time. Who was incarcerated? When were they incarcerated? And where were they incarcerated. Analyzing the data would be the next step.

The data from the chart shows the incarceration rate of different cultures and increasing the black male population over time.

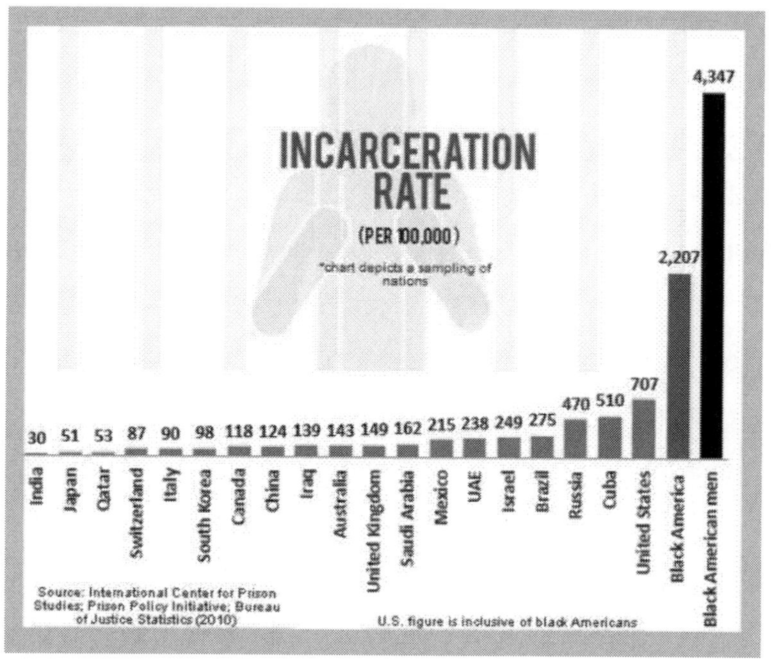


https://www.theatlantic.com/politics/archive/2014/10/mapping-the- new-Jim-crow/381617/

Before they look at possible solutions, they must ask the question why? Why are the number of black males going to prison increasing year after year? Research may reveal a variety of reasons for this epidemic. Ethics plays a critical role as it is a combination of laws, and policies that may affect the data. Systemic barriers are a combination of policies, rules, laws and treatment of specific groups of individuals that may continue to perpetuate a problem.

Does the incarceration rate of black males have a direct or indirect correlation to systemic barriers within our society? Do the laws in our society prepare a system for more black males to go to jail than any other sub-group of Americans? These are the questions we need to ask ourselves. After watching the documentary "13th Amendment" it seems as though the demographics of the prison population directly shows an increase number of African American men entering the prison system each year.

President Nixon carried his law and order campaign in which we began seeing an increase in the incarceration rate of black men. That number continued to increase over the years. President Bill Clinton introduced the "Three strikes you are Out Bill" which was to decrease crime on the streets of America. This mandatory "three strikes you are out law" did not decrease street crimes yet it allowed for a system to give mandatory minimum sentences for small crimes. It increased the long-term incarceration of the African American male population in prisons. This is an example of how ethics, may have played an essential role in the epidemic of black males in the prison population. Students can create their own solutions to help solve these problems. It allows students to utilize their critical thinking skills to become real world problem solvers. Presenting projects that will properly inform others of these problems. Making this information more available to students in minority and majority communities may give them a better chance of understanding the odds. As we see systemic barriers may affect a variety of epidemics. Students may begin to take interest into a career within the legal system. Others may be inspired to get more involved within the community to bring about awareness and change. After seeing my student's presentation of solutions to these problems, I would often think, if they can create solutions like this in a classroom what will they be able to do in the future?

**Human Trafficking**

Human trafficking has recently been named as one of the fastest growing epidemics affecting many families from various communities. The CDC recently added a division to collect data for human trafficking in 2018, which will record data for the fiscal year of 2019. CDC, information site.

Human trafficking is a serious topic and has increased as one of the most progressive crimes of choice in America over the past five years. It is a public health problem considered to be a form of modern-day slavery. The victims are working for the very same basic needs as slaves such as food, water and shelter. A common problem within several communities.

When someone is recruited to do forced labor by fraudulent means, he or she is a victim of human trafficking.

https://www.acf.hhs.gov/otip/about/what-is-human-trafficking

Teaching this topic to students in public schools would be something that could possibly increase their chances of survival within a complex world. Technology has provided both benefits and negative opportunities. Social media leaves little boundaries for our children and teenagers. History, analytics, descriptive, ethics, and public health surveillance solutions are the five areas that can be easily identified and studied when teaching human trafficking.

Students will find out that this is more of a global epidemic to say the least. A class such as this would include recent data from the CDC, bioinformatics, demographics, statistical analysis with current data and recent abductions. Students can once again design solutions to these problems with classroom discussions, speakers from law enforcement agencies and community leaders. The creativity and opportunity for real world application is limitless. Counselors and teachers may want to use the five frameworks as it gives a brief summary of the information categorized within a familiar concentration of knowledge. This unit allows for classroom or small discussions or individual counseling. The students can understand cause and effect. What causes an epidemic and what are the variables? What is the history of human trafficking and how far does this problem date back? What was the number of reported cases 20 years ago? What are the effects of modern technology on the human trafficking epidemic? This one topic provides several ideas for essential questions. Descriptive analyzes and identifies person, place and time. The demographics of the primary subgroup or victims from the epidemic are identified. Location includes detailed descriptions including, geographical location, race, gender, age, social and or cultural identity. Analytical epi would review the data and statistics. Types of research study designs along with the implementations for effective research. Ethics will build on the laws and policies enforced to decrease the number of victims. Stings, and stiffer penalties have been implemented over the past 5 years regarding sex trafficking. Surveillance of solutions and data allows one to create more effective strategies based on these different components.

**Infectious Diseases**

Infectious diseases have always been a major issue and may be one of largest threats to mankind. Humans have always had to deal with adversity, yet nothing has had the impact on man like infectious diseases. Infectious diseases are known to infect living organisms and may or may not be considered a living organism but utilizes a host to survive. These infections may be passed on by direct or indirect contact within a population. These diseases may be classified as viral, fungal, bacterial or protozoan infections. Sexually transmitted diseases are some of the most discussed and talked about within our society. Trichomonas, Syphilis and HIV are three different types of infections caused by organisms from various kingdoms and may not even be considered a living organism. Yet all are infections that have caused sickness and death throughout the world. Descriptive characteristics of sexually transmitted diseases seem to be greatest among African American women between the age of 15 to 24 years of age. Teenagers and younger Americans seem to be at the highest risk of exposure for such diseases. So “why would African American women be the largest subgroup with HIV and other sexually transmitted diseases. Several may not have access to good health care. Some may not be able to afford the co-pay to go to hospitals or local clinics. Furthermore, family traditions and habits may give some younger adults information on home remedies that may or may not be effective. Others may have old history stories of not always trusting the doctors from stories of the past. Nevertheless, HIV and other sexually transmitted disease continue to rise in the African American female population.

The Diagnosis of HIV among women in the US and Dependent Areas 2017

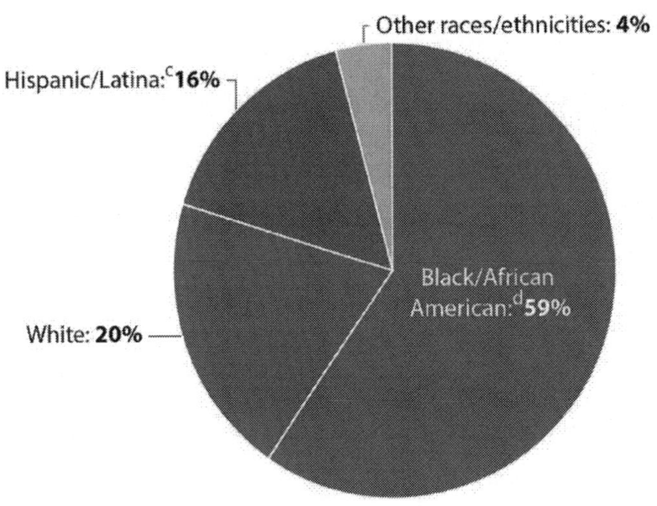


.

Using analytical data from confirmed cases, the CDC has provided a more descriptive breakdown of subgroups of HIV cases. Information such as this allows students to understand why some subgroups may be at a greater risk for catching specific diseases.

Other viruses may not only be spread by person to person contact but may be transmitted by a droplet spread. The droplet spread is created when someone with a virus sneezes or coughs within a specific environment. The common cold, Influenza Virus, and the Coronavirus are all viruses that may be spread by droplet spread. The average virus may travel several feet depending on the circulation of wind within an environment. It is at this time that a droplet spread may be able to contaminate someone near the source of the cough. Therefore, health officials urge distance communication during some severe infectious disease outbreaks. H1N1, SARS, Ebola and now Coronavirus have all given law makers reasons to mandate policies and laws aimed at reducing the spread of the outbreak. When studying the current Covid-19 outbreak, one may benefit by utilizing the five frameworks to discuss or explain all the parameters in solving a real-life outbreak. History gives a brief description of the morphology of the virus. How it affects the human body and how the body responds to Covid-19. Descriptive, which describes person, place and time allows scientist to evaluate and determine which subgroups are of the greatest risk for catching the virus. Recently we have heard several health care officials stress the safety and importance of those who are older and have a history of respiratory illness. It has also revealed that the origin was from Wuhan, China. Analytical shows the trend of the epidemic. The numbers of cases each day and how fast is the epidemic growing. Ethics involves the policies, laws, prevention interventions and how effective are these changes in creating a solution to decrease the spread of the infection. Most Americans are a little uncomfortable with the restrictions, yet it is a part of the overall solution to the problem. In order to defeat a virus, you must not give the virus an opportunity to spread. It can isolate itself within a host and spread to someone without showing signs in the host. This is what they mean by the words asymptomatic. Which means, a person may carry this virus and infect others without showing any signs of physical sickness. It is the responsibility of our political leaders to enforce laws to protect our overall population. Ethics is defined as a set of rules, laws and policies put in place by a specific society or culture. As the United States and several other countries undergo a state of emergency, several policies and laws have been temporarily put in place to ensure the safety of all. Reducing social interaction, requiring school closures while all employers are encouraged to allow employees the opportunity to work from home. Several of the professional and college sports organizations have cancelled or postponed events. None of us would have expected these things to be a part of our society in 2020. Yet currently it is a part of our reality. Public health surveillance of solutions allows the epidemiologist the opportunity to see if there is anything working that may show a turnover in numbers. Regarding Covid-19, Is there a decline in cases with the interventions that were put in place or do we need to provide new ones to contain the virus? Teaching these basic principles of public health in schools may give students the opportunity to truly adapt to a lifestyle that may help save their life and those they love the most. If we teach all students epidemiology and public health, we may allow them to understand the language, protocol and procedures for any public health emergency. Students becoming problem solvers should result in adults understanding how to deal with a real public health emergency. Today the Coronavirus or COVID-19 is a serious pandemic that has spread across the world. We understand some of its history. We see the descriptive of those most likely affected. Those with prior respiratory problems and senior citizens. We are currently watching the numbers go up each day. Currently killing more than 200,000 in the United States. No one would believe that during the year 2020 we would endure one of the most devasting infectious pandemics in our history, but it is now a reality. I hope we can all begin to understand the importance and value of teaching epidemiology and public health to all students. This may be a step in the direction for the change we need in order to teach our students adaptation skills. Before publishing this book, this morning, on October 2, 2020, I was informed that our current President of the United States, Donald J Trump and First Lady, Ivanka Trump tested positive for Covid-19. I wish them a speedy recovery as we each learn everyday how things can change within a moment's notice when it comes to an outbreak.

Teaching all humans how to survive a day longer is something worth learning. It may increase health awareness from a global perspective. Fredrick Douglass said it best, "It is easier to teach children, than try to change the mind of a grown man". We can do better as we see an ever-changing world taking those we so love at an elevated rate. We can change the future. Providing students, parents and community leaders, with relevant platforms that allows them to understand the pitfalls they may endure based on their own environment. Everyone can learn something new, from reducing infectious diseases, learning healthier eating habits, to behaviors that may prevent cancer. From mental illness to homicide there is a method for providing a clear breakdown of the problem in order to develop a solution. I have been afforded the opportunity to serve. To serve the purpose that was set for me since day one. We cannot solve every problem as humans; however, we can begin to educate our community one day at a time with one topic at a time. Educating a community on how to live a safer and healthier lifestyle is knowledge that breeds life. We can begin with our children and community tomorrow. Now more than ever, I believe we can all agree, that our country and world need LOVE.

# "Diamond in the Darkness"

GOD created the light from the darkness as energy for the creation of life and mankind. Any gifts that I have obtained, descend from that light. A diamond shines bright in the darkness. A diamond is also formed by a combination of carbon, pressure and time. My journey has not been short and has been developed over a period of more than 25 years. Throughout my journey I proudly live my life as a black man in the United States working in the field of education. I have also felt as though sometimes my light was dimmed by placing me in the closet. A closet full of darkness and sadness, yet somehow, I was able to continue shining my light. Only to realize the light was a reflection from the diamond within me. Within my dark brown skin ligaments, bones, muscles and heart, was a soul. A soul given the proper ingredients over time within the darkness producing a diamond. A diamond shining a light for everyone to see. Teaching epidemiology and public health to all people truly is my purpose and the diamond within my soul. I wrote this book to share to all, my Diamond in the Darkness.

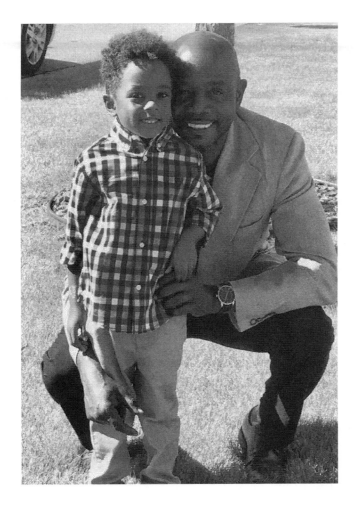

I want to thank all of those who have inspired, motivated and helped me continue to see the light within me. God, first and my mother Angelo Scott Williams and father the late Eddie V. Williams for bringing me into this world and providing me with the genes and light of life from above. My siblings, brothers Edward Williams, Eric Williams, Eddie Williams, sisters Linda Williams and Priscilla Williams. To my relatives in Montgomery, Alabama, Harvey Illinois, and Detroit Michigan. My colleagues from Jasper County Schools, Newton County Schools and Dekalb County School Districts in Georgia. Dr. Ralph Cordell, Dr. David Kleinbaum, Dr. Donna Stroup,

Dr. Rick Goodman, Dr. Ruth Berkelemen, Mr. Jimmy Jordan, Dr. Roderick Sams, Dr. Julian Cope, Mrs. Mary Lou Jordan, Dr. Craig Lockhart, Mr. John Ellenberg, Mr. Tracy Curtis, Mrs. Debbie Stephens, Mr. James Peek, Coach Robert Richardson, Mr. Jerry Williams, Coach Johnny Williams, Coach Jack Williams, Mr. Marcus Morris, Mr. Eric Arena, Dr. Sandra Owens, the late Dr. Charlene Davenport the late Dr. Stephen B. Thacker, the late Mr. Kenneth Daniels, the late Mr. Dan Arp and the late Mr. Mourad Eljourbagy. To all my friends and fraternity brothers of Alpha Phi Alpha, and Kappa Kappa Psi. My former and current colleagues in education and numerous associates. My thanks to all of you for making this book a part of your life.

May each one of you continue to have peace, LOVE and prosperity.

Evern Vinson Williams
Pioneer Science Teacher,

For more information go to www.loveforstudents.org

## Common Terms: Common Terms of Public Health and Epidemiology

**antibody-** Proteins in the blood used to fight microorganisms and infections in the body.

**association-** A relationship between two or more events or variables.

**attack rate** Measure of frequency of new cases of a health attack over a specific amount of time during an outbreak.

**attack rate, secondary-**Measurement of how often a new case or disease occurs.

**cause of disease-** Any event, object or variable that influences the spread of an infection or disease.

**clinical criteria-** Features of a disease that must be detected by a physician and or health care professional licensed to perform a clinical lab test.

**contagious -** The spread of a disease passed on by direct contact or proximity.

**determinant-** Variables or factors that brings about changes in the spread of an infection or disease on an environment.

**droplet spread-** Spreading by direct contact as a result of aerosol droplets being produced by coughing, sneezing, other form of spray.

**environmental factor-** All environmental factors that affect the rate at which an infection spread.

**Epidemic-** When an outbreak occurs over a large population smaller than global

**immunity, herd-** A specific groups ability to be resistant to a specific disease or infection.

**immunity, passive-** Immunity conferred by an antibody produced in another host. This type of immunity can be acquired naturally by an infant from its mother or artificially by administration of an antibody-containing preparation

**morbidity-** Disease; any departure, subjective or objective, from a state of physiological or psychological health and well-being.

**mortality rate-** A measure of the frequency of death in a defined population during a specified time interval.

**mortality rate, age-adjusted-** A mortality rate that has been statistically modified to account for the effect of different age distributions in different populations in a study.

**mortality rate, age-specific-** A mortality rate limited to an age group. In calculating age-specific mortality rates, the numerator is the number of deaths in the age group, and the denominator is the number of people in that age group.

**mortality rate, neonatal-** The mortality rate for children from birth up to, but not including 28 days of age. In calculating neonatal mortality rates, the numerator is the number of deaths in this age group during a given time period, and the denominator is the

number of live births reported during the period. The neonatal mortality rate is usually

expressed per 1,000 live births.

**mortality rate, osteomata-** The mortality rate for children from 28 days up to, but not including, 1 year of age. In calculating post neonatal mortality rates, the numerator is the number of deaths among this age group during a given time period, and the denominator is the number of lives births during the same period. The post neonatal mortality rate is usually expressed per 1,000 live births.

**mortality rate, race-specific-** A mortality rate limited to a specified racial group. Both numerator and denominator are limited to that group.

**mortality rate, sex-specific-** A mortality rate among either males or females.

**natural history of disease-** The course of a disease from the time it begins until it is resolved.

**notifiable disease-** A disease that, by law, must be reported to public health authorities upon diagnosis.

**Outbreak-** (*Syn: epidemic*) Because the public sometimes perceives "outbreak" as less sensational than "epidemic," it is sometimes the preferred word. Sometimes the two words are sometimes differentiated, with "outbreak" referring to a localized health

problem, and "epidemic," to one that takes in a more general area. (More at Epidemic).

**pandemic-** An epidemic occurring over a very wide area (several countries or continents) and usually affecting a large proportion of the population.

**population-** The total number of inhabitants of a given area or country. In sampling, the population may refer to the units, from which the sample is drawn, not necessarily the total population of people. A population can also be a group at risk, such as

**portal of entry-** A pathway into the host that gives an agent access to tissue that will allow it to multiply or act. Nasal, mucous membranes, and mouth.

**prevalence-** The number or proportion of cases or events or conditions in each population.

**Prevalence period-** The amount of a disease, or type of injury present in a population over a period.

**Rate-** An expression of the relative frequency with which an event occurs in a defined population.

**relative risk-** A comparison of the risk of a health problem in two groups.

**risk-** The probability that an individual will be affected by, or die from, an illness or injury within a stated time or age span.

**risk factor-** An aspect of personal behavior or lifestyle, an environmental exposure, or a hereditary characteristic that is associated with an increase in the occurrence of a disease, chronic condition, or injury.

**risk ratio-** A comparison of the risk of a health problem in two groups.

**sample-** A selected subset of a population. A sample may be random or nonrandom and representative or non-representative.

**sample, representative-** A sample whose characteristics correspond to those of the original or reference population.

**seasonality-** Change in physiological status or in the occurrence of a disease, chronic condition, or type of injury that conforms to a regular seasonal pattern.

**sensitivity-** The ability of a system to detect epidemics and other changes in the occurrence of health problems; the proportion of people with a health problem who are

correctly identified by a screening test or case definition. (See also Specificity).

**skewed-** A distribution that is asymmetrical.

**sporadic illness-** An illness that occurs infrequently and irregularly.

**study, experimental-** A study in which investigators identify the type of exposure that everyone (clinical trial) or community (community trial) has had and then follows the individuals' or communities' health status to determine the effects of the exposure.

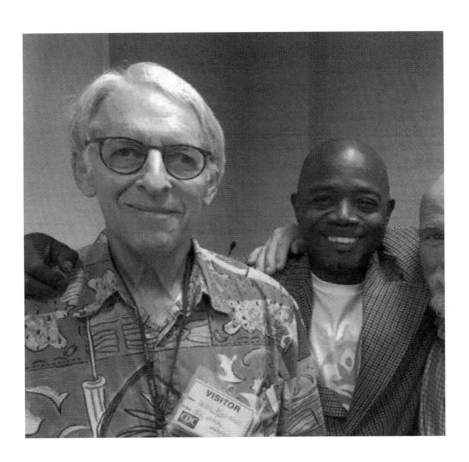

.

Made in the USA
Columbia, SC
03 August 2021

42900989R00115